"No matter what, we all get older. *Second Blooming* contains terrific information and a recipe to help women transcend the years after turning fifty."   —Deb Caruthers

"The authors provide encouragement and examples for women over fifty to challenge themselves with new and enriching opportunities, and avoid wasting time being miserable and stagnant. The book suggests engaging in new activities, acting spontaneously, and seizing moments of opportunity. I highly recommend this inspirational book for women entering their second blooming."   —Carol V. Allen, Ph.D.

"I have consistently observed, both in my personal life and in my practice as a geriatric physician, that the individuals who 'age successfully' are those who maintain a positive outlook on life. They have a purpose for being, and they value sharing their lives with others. They remain 'healthy' despite sometimes long lists of medical problems, disabilities, and multiple medications. *Second Blooming* can help them determine their purpose."   —Donna Jacobi, M.D.

"*Second Blooming* is THE guide for women over 50 looking to uncover and cultivate their talents, strengths, and skills as they embrace their 'second life.' Historic events of the 1960s and 1970s mean this is a transitional generation, with few role models. Luckily, *Second Blooming* opens a world of possibilities for a meaningful future in a culture that many times values youth and beauty over wisdom and experience. This book acts as a guide or personal coach, providing a step-by-step process for women to discover their purpose and decide how they want to spend their next decades."

—Jeff Nall, Editor-in-Chief, C   r *Seniors*

"We all have intrinsic values and gifts. We can use these gifts in unique ways, but developing them takes time, attention, and nurturing. We must never give up. At all ages and stages of life, we find the opportunity to serve. We are lifelong learners, but we need physical, mental, emotional, and spiritual stimulation to live well. *Second Blooming* helps women evaluate and assess where they are, then make an informed response to the question, *What do I want to do with the rest of my life?*"
—Jean Norman.

"Betsy and Kathleen know how to bloom! Learning from them how to put your best foot forward on this new journey of 'Life after 50' is learning from the masters. Their perennial bright spirits will take you to a new spring of your life, and a spring in your step. I highly recommend that you enjoy their perspective and take advantage of this opportunity for growth, renewal, and exciting life changes."
—Vicki Escude, author and Master Certified Coach

"For the past twelve years, I cared for my husband throughout his decline from Alzheimer's disease, and I grieved deeply after his death. I feel as if I didn't age normally, but just got old. I was confused by my change in status. I had lost my 'job' and my sense of direction. *Second Blooming* reminded me that I still have worth and is helping me uncover and redefine just what my dreams are. Now I feel that I can move forward and rediscover joy and purpose."   —Rochelle Kober.

"It's as if Kathleen and Betsy were living my life. Their insight into the new reality for women in their 50s is nothing less than astonishing. They offer a path that will guide and direct our new generation of women who are determined to bloom, and bloom again. With their help, we can and will find our green thumbs!"   —Pamela Bilbrey, author of *Ordinary Greatness: It's Where You Least Expect It...Everywhere.*

"I requested that Kathleen and Betsy write an article about "Second Blooming for Women" for my publication after hearing them speak at an American Business Women's Association meeting. The response to the article we ran was very positive. One of our readers wrote to us saying, "I just want to say how much 'Second Blooming' meant to me. I had just had my 70th birthday, and was really feeling a little old and a bit worthless. The article said to seek out your dreams and take action. Use your skills and take some risks. It encouraged me to forge ahead. I'm ready to take action, go for my dreams, and hope to make a difference. Thanks for reminding me that my life matters, regardless of age!!" We enjoy printing stories that really benefit our readers and this was in fact one of those articles." —Nancy Babin, Publisher, *On the Coast* magazine

"I look forward to using this book as a tool for the next phase of my life. The first phase, which spanned almost 30 years, consisted of being a military wife, a proud mother of one son, a Federal employee, and a dedicated daughter. In this next phase, I am divorced, childless, at the brink of retirement, and still a dedicated daughter. *Second Blooming* offers me a chance to rediscover the covered up parts of myself and assist me with my journey." —Sandye Cole.

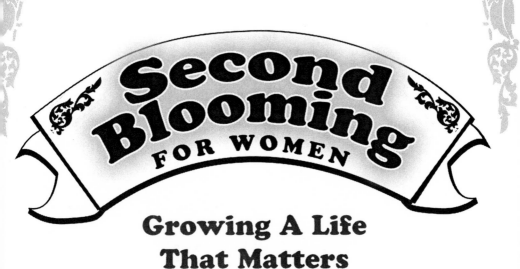

Second Blooming
FOR WOMEN

Growing A Life
That Matters
After Fifty

Kathleen Vestal Logan
E. L. (Betsy) Smith, Ph.D.

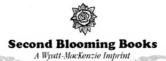

Second Blooming Books
A Wyatt-MacKenzie Imprint

Second Blooming for Women: Growing A Life That Matters After Fifty
by Kathleen Vestal Logan and E.L. (Betsy) Smith, Ph.D.

ISBN 978-0-9743832-5-5
Library of Congress Control Number:2009923979

Grateful acknowledgment is made to the following publishers for permission to quote copyrighted material:

The Southern Living Garden Book, edited by Steve Bender, Birmingham, Alabama: Oxmoor House, Inc., 1998, for flower descriptions of Texas sage, crabapple, lily, kudzu, rose, impatiens, and crepe myrtle.

Please Understand Me II: Temperament, Character, Intelligence by David Keirsey, Ph.D., Del Mar, California: Prometheus Nemesis Book Company, 1998, for quotes from and application of the Keirsey Temperament Sorter II (KTS-II).

From NEW PASSAGES by Gail Sheehy, copyright ©1995 by G. Merritt Corporation; Endpaper illustrations copyright ©1995 by Nigel Holmes. Used by permission of Random House, Inc.

Every effort was made to obtain permissions for material referenced in this book. If there are any concerns regarding the use of a quote or reference, please contact the publisher with your request.

We are also indebted to:
Shelby Miller for her previously unpublished poems.
Lyda Toy for original art work for each of the chapters.
Derek Ferebee for the cover photography.

www.secondbloomingforwomen.com

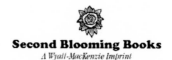

Second Blooming Books
A Wyatt-MacKenzie Imprint

Published by Second Blooming Books, A Wyatt-MacKenzie Imprint
Wyatt-MacKenzie Publishing, Inc.
15115 Highway 36, Deadwood, Oregon 97430
www.wymacpublishing.com

To our husbands
Jack Parkin and C. Flack Logan

And our mothers
Valeta Helberg Smith and Joan Marshall Vestal

"I have enjoyed greatly the second blooming that comes
when you finish the life of the emotions and
of personal relations; and suddenly find—at the age of fifty, say—that
a whole new life has opened before you."

~ Agatha Christie

C O N T E N T S

INTRODUCTION

Bloom where you're planted. Excellent advice, but it won't work for women over fifty because the landscape in which we were planted as girls or young women no longer exists. The entire environment changed in just one generation—ours—giving us the unprecedented opportunity to create and live a *Second Blooming.*

Background

This "second life" phenomenon has been explored by several women:

- Gail Sheehy published *New Passages: Mapping Your Life Across Time* in 1995. She maps a new frontier for people that she calls a "Second Adulthood" and concludes: "There is no longer a standard life cycle. People are increasingly able to customize their life cycles."[1]

- Sue Shellenbarger covers the consequences of a bad transition into life after fifty in *The Breaking Point,* published in 2005. She describes six modes of midlife crisis: sonic boom, moderate, slow burn, flameout, melt down, and non-starter. It's not hard to picture these, is it? Five are clearly troublesome, but she says, "A Moderate crisis entails less conflict and destruction…and may be the healthiest model of all."[2]

- Suzanne Braun Levine, first editor of *MS Magazine,* wrote the 2005 book *Inventing the Rest of Our Lives.* She expresses both the anticipation and angst many women feel, saying, "Second Adulthood is the unprecedented and productive time that our generation is encountering as we pass that dreaded landmark of a fiftieth birthday."[3]

- In her 2007 book, *Leap! What Will We Do with the Rest of Our Lives?,* Sara Davidson sums up the challenge we face: "There's a new life stage—after fifty and before eighty—and we're the ones whose mission it will be to figure out what to do with it."[4]

What we know, then, is that life after fifty is different for our generation; we can create a "second life" of our choosing; many of us fear getting older; and it's up to us to determine how best to use this stage of life.

The problem

Because we are a transitional generation, we can't look to older women as our models. We have decades yet to live, yet often feel marginalized in our youth-oriented culture. We're aware that time is limited, so we don't want to waste it. We also want to keep what is good and treasured from our lives so far while we create our future. How, then, can we minimize the pitfalls and maximize our opportunities?

Our solution

We wrote *Second Blooming* to help fill that need for guidance. Using our backgrounds in education, counseling, and coaching, we developed a model for a "moderate" mode of transition as suggested by Shellenbarger to assist women as they plan their lives after fifty. While many of the books we read were memoirs or stories about other women, we intend *Second Blooming* to be a book that lets you focus on *your* life.

As women who are cheerfully living our own *Second Blooming,* we want you to embrace this stage of life with optimism, too. This is a book to experience, not just to read, and with each chapter, we'll coach you toward growing a life that matters.

What to expect in the book

Part I is *Gardening 101—Know Your Environment.* This section will help you understand the historical context in which our generation grew up, and what impact it had on you. It then takes a frank look at the perceived woes and often-unexpected joys of growing older. An open attitude and a willingness to change are proposed as necessary ingredients for growing.

Part II is *Do a Soil Analysis—Know Yourself.* These are exciting chapters of self-exploration and revelation. First, you'll identify "weeds" in your life, common behaviors that can inhibit your potential. Chapter 6 addresses the critical importance of self-trust. In chapters 7 and 8, you'll identify your personality type, as well as the specific talents, strengths, and skills you already possess which will give direction and focus to your choices.

Part III is *Be a Master Gardener—Grow Yourself.* In these final chapters, you'll take everything you've learned about yourself so far and use it to decide which passions and dreams you want to cultivate. Step-by-step, you'll create a plan for your *Second Blooming.*

Getting the most out of the book

This isn't a book to dash through; instead, savor each chapter. You may find the need to stop now and then to absorb newfound knowledge, so allow yourself that interlude. Since this is a life change you're considering, it's well worth the investment of time and thought. You may want to work through this book with a friend or friends who are also ready to make the transition.

As you'll note, we took turns writing different chapters. Also, we held conversations frequently with a small group of women of various ages who contributed their perspectives. They enrich the book, and the sharing process itself was uplifting to all of us. What a grand chance to take the long view of our lives while encouraging and supporting each other. By the time you finish the book, you may feel like they're your friends, too. They include Deb, 52; Beth, 57; Maripaul, 59; Mary, 61; Mamie, 61; Shirley, 63; Shelby, 69; and Anne, 85.

Have a journal or notebook with you when you read so you can keep all of your thoughts and findings in one spot. At the end of each chapter, you'll find activities to enhance and expand your experience, or apply new skills and knowledge. Additional reading resources are given if you want to learn more about the subject. Also, look at the flower sketch at the beginning of the chapter to see if you can determine why we chose that particular flower to illustrate that particular topic. It's a tiny botanical mystery to consider.

Seize the chance

Joan Anderson, author of *The Second Journey: The Road Back to Yourself,* believes the "second journey" begins when change is thrust upon you, creating a crisis of feelings.[5]

However, we don't believe it's necessary for you to experience a crisis to take advantage of this favorable combination of circumstances. Certainly, for some, there may be death or divorce or an event that precipitates action, but we encourage all women to seize this chance, to anticipate life after fifty instead of passively reacting to it or letting it slip away. Everyone asks the essential questions: "Why am I here? Does my life matter?" Living a life of significance doesn't happen by accident; instead, it must be cultivated with conscious, thoughtful choices.

Your *Second Blooming* isn't guaranteed, though, and could be stunted by a lack of nurturing, a "late freeze," or an unwillingness to grasp the chance. Yes, you're growing older, but why not also grow bolder? Why not make this time of your life *the* time of your life? Your life is your garden, utterly unique, and you are the head gardener. With each chapter, you'll see more clearly the direction of your own garden path, and start walking it with confidence, anticipation, and excitement.

Our promise to you

By being actively involved in *Second Blooming*, we promise you will:

- understand why you have this historic opportunity
  for a *Second Blooming*;
- claim your personality, talents, and strengths;
- identify your skills;
- clarify your passions, dreams, and values;
- build confidence and self-trust;
- know what your options are for the future;
- create your life purpose statement;
- design a plan to translate your purpose into action.

It's time to start

This book is your personal almanac for growing a life that matters after fifty, so dig in. Get ready to bloom where you plant yourself.

Part I

Gardening 101
Know Your Environment

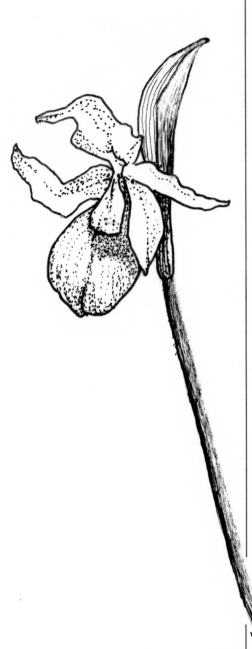

Lady's Slipper

Lady's slippers are found living in open fens, bogs, swamps, and damp woods where there is plenty of light. They grow slowly, taking up to sixteen years to produce their first flowers. Plants live up to fifty years and grow four feet tall. A century ago, the lady's slipper was a favorite adornment on rural church altars during the summer.

— *State of Minnesota Web site*

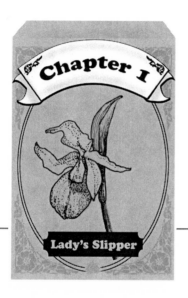

Chapter 1

Lady's Slipper

History Sows the Seeds for Women's Second Blooming

by Kathleen

"There is a revolution in the life cycle. In the space of one short generation the whole shape of the life cycle has been fundamentally altered."
~ Gail Sheehy

A subset of your husband. That's how you would have been seen in the early 1800s, and your job was to be obedient to him. Even if you had property or money, it became his upon your marriage. You had no legal rights, were not entitled to voice independent thoughts or opinions in public, and certainly had no right to vote. Education wasn't an option because "intense physical or intellectual activity would be injurious to the delicate female biology and reproductive system."[1] So much for the good old days.

Two hundred years later, men and women have equal rights under the law, and you can create a life of your own choosing after age fifty, a "second life." What happened?

Betsy and I asked several women, "In your lifetime, what were the most significant historical events for women?" They chose just a few, which sowed the seeds of opportunity for women's *Second Blooming*. As you read about them below, look for themes of change in laws, attitudes, culture, and reproduction. Think, too, about which of these changes required more time for their full impact to take effect.

Seed 1: The right to vote

"Remember the Ladies," Abigail Adams implored in a letter to her husband, John, who was working on the Declaration of Independence in 1776. Much as Adams valued his wife, the Declaration specified only "all men are created equal."[2]

Much later, in 1840, Elizabeth Cady Stanton and Lucretia Mott went to London to attend the World Anti-Slavery Convention. Furious at being sent to sit in the balcony as observers because they were women, they returned home resolved to hold their own convention. Stanton prepared and presented her Declaration of Principles, including Resolution 9, requesting the right to vote. In 1848, the first women's rights convention was held in Seneca Falls, New York, where many participants signed a Declaration of Sentiments and Resolutions, outlining the main issues and goals for the nascent women's suffrage movement.[3]

Stanton, Sojourner Truth, Susan B. Anthony, and other women worked tirelessly during the Civil War for the emancipation of slaves, believing that both slaves and women would be granted the same rights afterwards. But for political reasons, suffrage for African Americans and women was separated, with President Lincoln saying, "This hour belongs to the Negro."[4]

Women persisted, despite setbacks. The 14th Amendment to the Constitution, ratified in 1868, "defined 'citizenship' and 'voters' as 'male,' and raised the question as to whether women were considered citizens of the United States at all."[5] Although the 15th Amendment in 1870 enfranchised black men, women were still excluded. Susan B. Anthony pushed the issue by trying to vote for Ulysses S. Grant for president in 1872, an act for which she was arrested and sent to trial.[6]

In 1878, the Woman Suffrage Amendment was finally introduced in the United States Congress, but it was forty-two more years before it was ratified as the 19th Amendment in 1920.[7] Stanton, Anthony, Truth, and many other women who had worked so hard to secure the right to vote for women died before they could exercise that right.

Looking at my own family, my grandmothers would have been the first women to be able to vote, my mother second, and I would be only the third generation. Who do you think were the first women in your family to vote?

Seed 2: The Pill

My Grandmother Marshall bore fourteen children, two of whom died. My mother had five children, with at least one miscarriage, giving birth to my youngest "surprise" brother when she was forty-two, a decade after her fourth child had been born. Birth control was unreliable, at best, for the generations of women who preceded us.

In fact, "History reveals that before the development of The Pill, women tried a variety of 'nature's elixirs' as contraceptive methods. They drank mercury, swallowed carrot seeds, ingested diluted copper ore, or drank a brew of beaver testicles soaked in alcohol."[8] Yum. A little more palatable, diaphragms and condoms had been available since the 1840s. By 1951, the Catholic Church had broadened its views, sanctioning the rhythm method of birth control in addition to abstinence.

Margaret Sanger, who established the Planned Parenthood Federation, actually envisioned the birth control pill in 1912; she was arrested in 1916 for opening the country's first birth control clinic.[9] But it wasn't until 1951, at age 72, that Sanger managed to help secure funds to instigate medical research for the Pill project.[10] In 1957, Enovid was approved by the Food and Drug Administration (FDA) for the treatment of severe menstrual disorders; the drug's label noted a "side effect" of preventing ovulation.[11]

Not surprisingly, by 1959, "an unusually large number of American women mysteriously develop[ed] severe menstrual disorders and ask[ed] their doctors for the drug."[12] Enovid was officially approved for sale as an oral contraceptive in 1960, and for the first time in history, women had reliable control over their reproductive biology. Other changes also had to occur because as late as 1961, for example, it was still a crime to use birth control in Connecticut.[13]

By 1965, 6.5 million American women were taking the Pill, making it the most popular form of reversible birth control. Ten million women were using it by 1973. With a new ability to manage childbearing, women began entering the workforce in increasing numbers, with 60% of American women of reproductive age employed by 1982.[14] "No longer forced into motherhood by their biology, women could choose how they wanted to shape their lives, planning when to have children and how many to have. Meanwhile, they could pursue higher education and careers."[15]

The entire culture had to shift to accommodate women's new roles.

What impact did the Pill's development have on your life? On other women you know? What changes did you observe in our culture as a result of the Pill?

Seed 3: The Feminine Mystique

I was a junior in college in 1963 when Betty Friedan published *The Feminine Mystique*, in which she made the radical proposal that men and women were created equal, and attacked the notion that women could only find fulfillment through childbearing and homemaking. She said, "The fact that American women are kept from growing to their full human capacities is taking a far greater toll on the physical and mental health of our country than any known disease."[16]

Coupled with the expanding use of the Pill, Friedan's book had an immediate and controversial impact on America, setting off the women's movement, or "women's lib," as many of us called it. We were participants, ready or not, in the forces her book unleashed. As Friedan observed, "By 1970, it was beginning to be clear that the women's movement was more than a temporary fad, it was the fastest growing movement for basic social and political change of the decade."[17] When Friedan died in 2006, a *New York Times* article said, "Rarely has a single book been responsible for such sweeping, tumultuous and continuing social transformation."[18]

Friedan was a leader of the feminist movement, co-founding the National Organization for Women (NOW), which was concerned with issues of childcare, abortion rights, equality, and representation in government. She lived to be 85, publishing her last book *The Fountain of Age* in 1993.

Only in preparing to write this book did I read *The Feminine Mystique*, which I found surprisingly relevant to life after fifty. Did you ever read it? If so, did it have any impact on you?

Seed 4: Civil Rights Act of 1964

Sometimes a man can get too clever. Howard W. Smith of Virginia chaired the House Rules Committee when the act was proposed and was opposed to civil rights laws for blacks. Alice Paul, a women's rights leader since 1917, urged him to add gender to the list of protected categories (race, color, religion, or national origin) in the bill. As a joke, he did add "sex," believing it would get the bill defeated. The joke backfired, and the monumental Civil Rights Act of 1964 was passed.[19]

The act was first proposed by President Kennedy in 1963, but was highly contentious. However, President Johnson signed an even stronger version into law on July 2, 1964, "following one of the longest debates in Senate history."[20] The various pieces of the act are called titles and, briefly, some of the more significant ones did the following:[21]

- Title I barred unequal application of voter registration require-ments;
- Title II outlawed discrimination in hotels, motels, restaurants, theaters, and all other public accommodations engaged in inter-state commerce;
- Title III encouraged the desegregation of public schools;
- Title VI prevented discrimination by government agencies that receive federal funding;
- Title VII outlawed discrimination in employment in any business on the basis of race, color, religion, sex, or national origin.

Originally conceived to protect the rights of black people, the bill as amended included women *for the first time.* This was a huge step forward for women in general, but especially for black women who benefited from both race and gender rights. Title VII specifically provided for equal employment opportunities in the workplace. "There was an immediate and highly visible increase in the numbers of women and minority group members who gained employment in the nation's factories and offices. The workforce in the United States, particularly the highly skilled and professionalized workforce, went from being predominantly white male to having substantially increased proportions of women and minorities."[22]

Laws extending civil rights to all Americans now existed. In your experience, how quickly did you notice changes in attitudes as a result of the Civil Rights Act? Did job opportunities change? There was also violence as people claimed their rights; were you affected by any?

Seed 5: Title IX

Eight years later, in 1972, Title IX of the Education Amendments to the Civil Rights Act of 1964 was passed. It covered many areas of public schooling, such as course offerings, admissions, and education programs, but athletics has received the most attention. The impact has been significant: "In 1972, when Title IX became law, fewer than 32,000 women played sports in college and fewer than 300,000 girls in high school. Helped by Title IX, those numbers have risen to more than 170,000 women and more than three million girls" according to a May 2008 article.[3]

Although the goal was to create parity in athletic opportunities and quality for males and females, controversy again erupted as many saw the emergence of girls' and women's athletics as draining funds from long-established boys' and men's sports. Tension continues, as seen in a recent lawsuit. When two female coaches at Fresno State, California "questioned school administrators about what they viewed as inequities in staffing, facilities, and job demands between the men's and women's athletics programs," they were fired. The women went to court alleging sex discrimination; separate juries sided with the women in 2007.[24] The university has appealed the decision.

Of special interest, sexual harassment was designated as a prohibited form of sex discrimination under Title IX, protecting both students and teachers.[25] As a whole, Title IX ensured that girls and women could have equal opportunities in education and sports, free from sexual harassment. Both their minds and bodies could grow and become strong.

What effect, if any, did Title IX have on your ability to participate in athletic activities? How did boys and young men view girls and young women who enjoyed athletics?

Seed 6: Roe v. Wade

There's no need to tell you what a troublesome issue abortion remains in our lives and politics. Nevertheless, let's look at the factual history. "When America was founded, abortion was legal. Laws prohibiting abortion were introduced in the mid1800s, and by 1900 most had been outlawed. Outlawing abortion did nothing to prevent pregnancy."[26] States began liberalizing laws in the 1960s, when civil rights and women's movements were underway. Or perhaps government's intrusiveness into family life had gone too far, for in 1965, the Supreme Court "struck down laws that banned the sale of condoms to married people" and thereby established a "right to privacy" in Griswold v. Connecticut.[27]

Eight years later in 1973, the Supreme Court ruled in Roe v. Wade that "during the first trimester, a woman has the right to decide what happens to her body."[28] The Court based its decision on the "right to privacy" established in the Griswold case.

Grassroots efforts to ban all abortions took an especially nasty turn in the 1990s. Here in Pensacola, for instance, two doctors who worked at women's clinics were murdered, as was a volunteer escort. Nationally, tensions are still high and legal challenges to Roe v. Wade remain active.

Whatever your personal belief, abortion, along with the Pill and other improved birth control options, provided women significant control over childbearing.

How old were you when Roe v. Wade was passed? What impact, if any, did the law have on your life or on the lives of your friends? What is your position on Roe v. Wade?

Impact of the seeds that were planted

Altogether, the tumultuous events of the 1960s and 1970s mean we are tilling new ground as a transitional generation. As girls, most of us were raised for traditional roles, then as adults lived lives quite different than we anticipated. We (especially those of us over sixty) started out to become homemakers, nurses, teachers, or secretaries, but often veered into new fields as laws gave us equality. Now we find ourselves, decades later, poised to take advantage of the bounty of the seeds sown by history for our *Second Blooming*.

As a group, those of us over fifty will live longer than previous generations, are healthier, have more money, are better educated, can access a virtual world with computers, have built a wide variety of skills, and are accustomed to planning our own lives. But there are few models or guidelines for us, so we'll have to create them as we go. Floundering after retirement, one friend muttered, "I need a guidance counselor, like the kids have in high school." It's a little like growing up in a desert, then spending maturity in a tropical garden. Different, challenging, exhilarating.

Now that you've had an overview of the changed landscape, you'll learn about women's "growing zones" in the next chapter and the meaningful life you can have if you embrace the potential.

ACTIVITIES

Put an X on the timeline when you were born. Were you born before, during, or after most of the historic events? What difference, if any, did that make? Which event(s) had the most significance for you and your life choices?

History Sows the Seeds for Women's *Second Blooming*

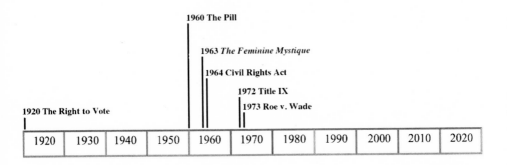

Write your own life story. Don't worry about errors, eloquence, or length; just think back to what was happening in your life and jot down your memories.

You can read Betsy's and my life stories and how our lives were changed by history on our Web site www.secondbloomingforwomen.com.

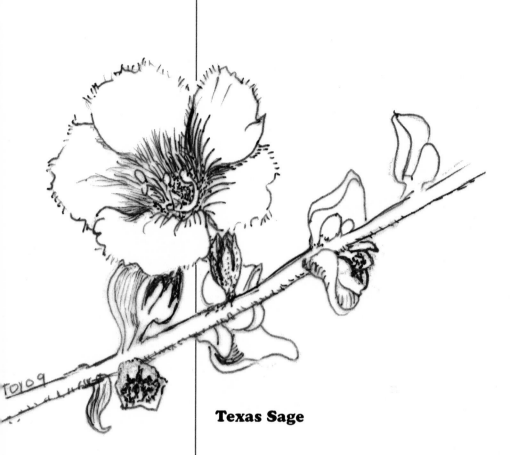

Texas Sage

Texas sage is native to the Southwest and northern Mexico. These compact, slow-growing shrubs are highly useful and attractive in dry, chalky soils. Most have silvery foliage and a good show of open bell-shaped flowers. They tolerate wind and heat, but often fail in high-rainfall, high-humidity areas.

— *The Southern Living Garden Book, 273*

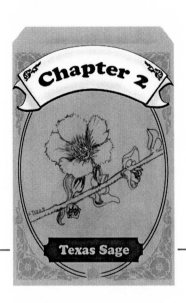

Chapter 2

Texas Sage

Climate Map: Thrive in Your Natural Growing Zone

by Kathleen

"The most notable fact that culture imprints on women is the sense of our limits. The most important thing one woman can do for another is to illuminate and expand her sense of actual possibilities." ~ Adrienne Rich

Texas sage comes from Betsy's home state, growing best in dry, chalky soils. If she tries to plant some in hot and humid Florida, it will surely die. Just as plants thrive best in their natural climate, so will you, agewise. You can keep pretending you're forty-nine, but it's gone forever, and aren't you smarter today anyway? Life for women over fifty is full of joyful opportunities, but many are unaware of the possibilities and potential because it's unexplored new territory. Perhaps, I thought, if women could see what life after fifty *could* be, they would embrace it rather than try to avoid it. The Women's Growing Zones chart that follows is the result.

As children, we're egocentric, certain that we are the center of our universe. Other people exist to serve and love us. We have an incredible capacity for learning, and everything fascinates us, from tiny sand crabs at the beach to changes in the shape of the moon.

When we become adults, we take on more responsibilities—at work, building a career, perhaps becoming a wife and mother. We're more practical, making decisions with our heads rather than our hearts. These are the "responsible" years, which we often spend nurturing others. Our mantra becomes "I have to" instead of a child's "I want to." What we do in our middle decades is necessary and normal for that time of life, but often our sense of self becomes buried under daily pressures, demands on our time, and the needs of other people.

Accept your natural growing zone

After fifty, life continues to shift focus. Look at Zone 3. Once again, like a child, you can be yourself, only magnified by all of your experiences and wisdom. If you allow yourself to move into your age's natural growing zone, bountiful opportunities await you. These are purposeful years, and your new mantra will become "I choose to."

Women's Growing Zones

Zone 1	Zone 2	Zone 3
Baby/child Selfish "I want to"	Adult woman Responsible "I have to"	Woman after 50 Purposeful "I choose to"
World is wide open; no focus	Building career and family	World expands again; focused
Self-oriented	Other-oriented	World or community-oriented
World exists to serve me	Give my best to others; little personal freedom, many responsibilities	Living an authentic life, using talents, strengths, skills for something meaningful
Sense of entitlement	Personal dreams put on hold, buried or forgotten, not a priority	My dreams are unearthed; I'm serving, contributing my gifts to world or community
Wildly expanding knowledge and abilities	Respond to external demands; many activities to juggle	Fewer, but more meaningful, activities and commitments
Use sensory experiences	Focus on head; rational and practical	Follow heart, soul, passions
Open to love from all sources	Love family, friends	Love of humanity
Yes and no clearly expressed	Often unsure when, why, or how to say yes and no	Yes and no are tied to my goals and values
Feelings are transparent	Feelings are suppressed or masked	I own my feelings, value myself, live true to my nature
Developing an identity, a sense of self	Sense of "self" gets lost or put aside	Living my purpose; clear sense of self; freedom to choose
It's always my turn	Will I ever get a turn?	It's my turn again to rekindle my passions and dreams
Life lasts forever; death has no meaning	Death is real, but distant	Death is real and getting closer, but motivating
No time limits on life	There's always tomorrow	It's now or never

Since moving from one zone to the next happens gradually, highlight on each line of the chart (moving left to right) which of the three phrases best describes you today. If you prefer, you can print the chart from our Web site: www.secondbloomingforwomen.com.

In general, you'll have marks in Zones 2 and 3 (although one frustrated woman said, "My sister's age is in Zone 3, but her behavior's stuck in Zone 1.").

The goal of this book is to help you steadily advance into Zone 3 so you can reap its benefits. It's time to rejoice in being alive, and like all plants and flowers, you'll bloom most brilliantly in your natural climate.

If the benefits of living in Zone 3 are so significant, what holds us back? Several cultural forces are at work that we need to be aware of, so let's start by being honest about the issues women face as we get older.

Society's view of older women

Betsy and I asked our women's discussion group, "How does our society view women over fifty?" which prompted various responses. Shelby said, "I do see the negatives. The pictures presented in fashion, on TV—they're young women with big lips and eyes, they're thin—they look like what we're "supposed" to. Even older men don't notice me anymore. No heads turn when I walk in a room. The conversation is directed toward younger people." Then she added, "My husband keeps reinforcing for me how attractive I am, but he has a young mental picture of me."

Beth didn't agree with the negative picture many women have. "I view women over fifty as beautiful, gifted. I personally don't see negativity based on age or a loss of value. Beauty is superficial. Looks have never driven me, except in my teens."

Maripaul observed, "As more women of notoriety become fifty, it's changing somewhat. But there's still a bias against older women."

Mary added, "Society may not be supportive of women our age, but we can ride the top of the wave with affirmations from our husbands and friends."

"I predict boomers will change society," said Beth. "We're going to force new options, creative alternatives. As a group, we're large, powerful, smart."

Since Deb had recently turned fifty, I asked her if she'd started feeling invisible yet, as so many of us do. She was emphatic. "Absolutely. Every woman alive knows exactly what you mean about turning invisible after fifty. It's painful."

Health issues

"What's hard about getting older?" we also asked. Shelby immediately responded, "Health. My sister, for example, just found out she has Parkinson's. Health limits what resources you can use for a full life."

Mary agreed. "When I was diagnosed with lupus, my pain was so severe, I wasn't sure I could continue. At best, I figured I could live for two years."

For Maripaul, "The biggest thing for me now is always being in pain. I can't do what I really enjoy, like surfboarding. Since I wasn't going to be a physically active retired person, I had to change my focus."

While such big health concerns can stop us in our tracks, most of us live as well as we can within our physical limits.

Impact of losing our jobs

Other losses come with aging, too. Whether by choice or necessity, many of us leave our jobs. For years, that job provided not only money, but also relationships, status, security, and a sense of self. For women whose self-image is totally wrapped up in the job, this loss can be devastating. When I first met Mary, lupus had forced her to take a leave of absence from teaching, and she spent the first year just trying to enhance her health. Feeling considerably better after two years, she had to decide whether or not to return to the classroom. Her doctor advised against it, and she reluctantly concurred. But then she faced another huge loss— her self-image—because, "I was born to be a second grade teacher. When I couldn't teach anymore, I felt empty. The teacher part of me was pulled out and there was nothing left. I questioned, *Who am I?*"

When Beth's husband developed life-threatening cancer, they sold their home in San Diego and moved into a small beach house he had owned for decades in Pensacola Beach, Florida. A navy wife, Beth was accustomed to moving, but this time she had to leave a job she loved. "Letting go of my career was the hardest part. I went through a period of despair, wondering, *Who am I?*"

Mary and Beth had both asked themselves a version of the existential questions, "Why do I exist? Does my life matter?" Each one of us must answer the questions for ourselves by the choices we make in our lives. It's harder than you'd think, since society seems to tell us that when we're older, it's acceptable and even desirable to follow the pleasure principle, to live the rest of our lives without purpose or meaning. Don't worry about fulfillment or value or authenticity. Play golf! Have fun! Be happy! Maripaul says the message to women is, "You're done. Be quiet. Go enjoy your grandchildren."

Don't misunderstand: Betsy and I encourage you to have fun, to enjoy simple pleasures, to play with your grandchildren; it's essential. But despite what society implies, you can also live on another level, a purposeful one, which is gratification of a different kind.

Losing family and friends

I look at the obituary page now, acutely aware that my age group is "moving up." When my mother died in 1994, I recall vividly a feeling of being eyeball-to-eyeball with eternity because there was no longer a parent in line ahead of me. Yet as parents, we do want to keep the natural order of life. I chuckle to remember my mother in a wheelchair looking at my brother in his wheelchair just two months before she died, saying, "I want to die before you do, and you don't look so good." She did, and he passed away only four months later.

Friends, too, are beginning to die. Friends are a special blessing in life, helping us to live fully, endure our pains and losses, and celebrate our joys. They are our family by choice, each irreplaceable. "I hear that from my mom," agreed Mary. "She's ninety-four and when she looks at pictures, almost everyone in them is gone. Maybe what it suggests is that we need a mix of ages in our lives."

Losing your spouse is documented to be the biggest source of stress, requiring you to redefine yourself and your place in the world. You never "get over it," but must instead live with it and through it, eventually creating a new "normal" for yourself.

Our bodies, our looks

Ah, yes, there's that other great loss, reserved especially for women: our youthful good looks. Don't you wonder when those age spots arrived on your hands? And those lines and bags around your eyes? Or why it's so hard to lose those pesky extra pounds? It seems every spring when the weather warms that my body has done naughty things under my winter clothes—sagging upper arms, rounder tummy, thighs bumpy with cellulite.

Decades ago, women used to be able to "age gracefully," but now we're expected to look forever young, using whatever means necessary. And the means are expanding all the time. Glance in any women's magazine and you'll see lots of ads for breast enlargement or reduction, nose or chin surgery, tummy tucks, and brow lifts. You can treat heavy eyelids, sagging jowls, smile lines (what's wrong with them?), and furrowed brows, thinning lips, and ropy necks. Treatment methods vary from surgery, to Botox and injectable fillers, to microdermabrasion and laser. But the message is consistent: You *are* your body, and your body isn't good enough. Change it. Fix it. Look young. One plastic surgeon takes this to the extreme with an ad for his services picturing a headless woman.

Check it out for yourself by looking in some women's magazines. Who is pictured? What ages do they seem to be? How do they look? How many seem to be over fifty? What kinds of ads *do* feature older women? For what products? What seems to be the media's unwritten message to older women?

When you buy into the notion that you are only a body, you lose. When you wish or pretend to be younger, you deny reality—who you *really* are—and you miss the opportunity to plan and flourish in maturity. You lose perspective on life itself, that you are part of a process that is ever-changing and ever-intriguing. You are so much more than just a body; you are a grown woman, full of life and dreams yet to be fulfilled, and age gives you the experience and wisdom to live abundantly. As Mary said, "We have so much more to be beautiful about. Our lives have been enriched by our years."

Here's the bottom line: Are you going to keep trying to buy into the illusion that you can and must look forever young? Or are you going to face reality by accepting yourself as a whole person—body, mind, and soul—and get on with being the best possible woman you can be, whatever your age? It's your choice.

The "good" losses

There are losses in life after fifty, but they're not all bad. I realized as I was writing this chapter that I had experienced many positive ones. Here are some for which I am grateful:

- Fear of failure. I have lost my fear of failure, which allows me to write this book. I'm willing to take the risk because I believe in what Betsy and I are doing, no matter how daunting the process.

- Aversion to risk. Recently, for example, I entered a Toastmasters speech contest. I gave the seven-minute speech with no notes, which had always provided security even if I never looked at them. The risk, of course, was having my mind go completely blank, which happened the first time I made the speech. Had I been age thirty, I'd have cried and quit, but I persisted.

- Shyness. I was abysmally shy well into my thirties and even forties. I'm still basically a quiet person, but I can now confidently fill leadership position, speak to groups of people, and hold lively seminars. And when I enter a room, I automatically look for whoever is standing alone and introduce myself because I know what it's like to be an introvert and overlooked.

- Job. I no longer have a full-time job, which affords me time for piano lessons, book and writing groups, walking and exercising with my husband, long-postponed trips, volunteer work, and especially writing this book. I have time for my choices.

- Family responsibilities. While I grieved deeply when my mother died, her death also freed me from the enormous stress of managing her rapidly declining health while working full time. Our son, too, is grown and gone, with a wonderful wife and an adorable daughter. My only job now is to love them and visit when possible.

- Lack of focus. I'm no longer scattered, pulled in a dozen directions. Little by little, I've ended multiple commitments and responsibilities, focusing on what I want to do and accomplish.

- Forever. This is the most significant loss. At my age, I'm well aware that time is limited, that I won't live forever. It makes me think, choose, prioritize, and do. There's no time to procrastinate if I ever want to say, "I'm making a difference. My life matters."

What's good about growing older?

Betsy and I posed this question to the women, too, and there was a variety of positive responses. Shelby said, "I'm much more outgoing. I can approach people. Before, I was much more reserved. I feel free to express my opinion. I'm open to meeting new people."

Beth said, "I'm *so* seeking opportunities! I'm impervious to magazines. It's time to just choose what I want."

"What's best is having the freedom to choose how to spend time," agreed Mary. "And the pleasure in family, kids and grandkids, of having an impact on them."

While writing this book, we heard stories from many women. One felt more capable because she organized a fund-raiser, which was quite successful, something she said she couldn't have done when she was younger. Other women valued being able to do what they knew was right without worrying about the impact on their career. And most had lost the need to be liked by everyone; instead, they were more content with themselves and chose to be with people who valued them.

A sense of urgency, because life's clock is ticking, helps us to not waste time on things that aren't important to us. We also largely possess by now the skills, confidence, and attitudes that allow us to be both productive and fulfilled. As Beth observed, "Youth was the time to gather our tools; now is the time to use them."

The new reality for women over fifty

We will live longer than previous generations of women, but will we live better? That question is posed in *Younger Next Year for Women* by Chris Crowley and Henry S. Lodge, M.D. Lodge is an internal medicine doctor and Crowley is both his patient and co-author already in his seventies. They caution, "Americans have achieved such staggering longevity that the real problem is outliving the quality of life, not running out of quantity."[1]

Crowley and Dr. Lodge then reassure us with "two amazing numbers, right up front: 70 percent of aging, for women as for men, is voluntary…you do not have to do it. And you can also skip 50 percent of all the sickness and serious accidents you'd expect to have from the time you turn fifty to the day you die."[2] Wonderful! Not only will we live longer, but also we can live healthier and better, or, in other words, *functionally younger.*

The keys they identify? Just three: exercise, nutrition, and commitment. Their book covers the first two but just touches on commitment, which our book covers in depth. All the work you do and plans you make are for nothing if your body fails you, so start building a healthy physical foundation today for your *Second Blooming.*

Medical advances have given us bonus years, and history has provided us a huge landscape of opportunities. The next step is up to each one of us. What will *you* do? Accept society's notion that older makes you less valuable, and limit your options accordingly? Or treasure yourself, your passions and dreams, and choose to live purposefully and abundantly?

You can start by preparing the soil of your life's garden—your attitude—in the next chapter.

ACTIVITIES

Talk with an older woman whom you respect. Ask such questions as: How have women's lives and opportunities changed in your lifetime? What's hard or challenging about getting older? What's good? If you could give a word of advice to women about aging, what would it be?

Are any women you know obsessed with losing their looks? How do they try to stave off the aging process? What's the cost to them of focusing so intently on the body?

What "good losses" have you experienced that have helped to prepare you for your Second Blooming?

RESOURCES

New Passages: Mapping Your Life Across Time by Gail Sheehy.

Younger Next Year for Women: Live Strong, Fit, and Sexy—Until You're 80 and Beyond by Chris Crowley and Henry S. Lodge, M.D.

Crabapple

Crabapple is a small, usually tart apple. Many kinds are valued more for their spring-time flowers than for their fruit; these are flowering crabapples. Some selections are used for jelly making and pickling. Other crabapples are prized for cider.

— *The Southern Living Garden Book, 195*

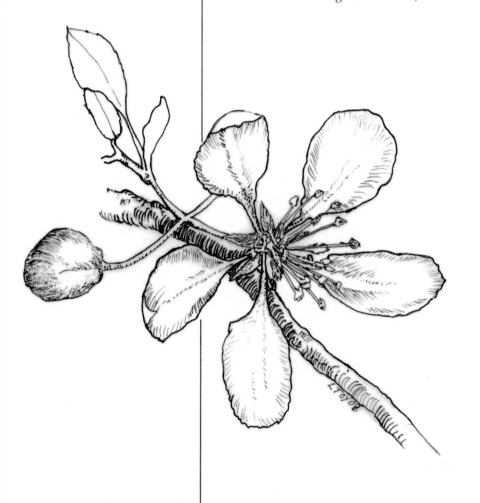

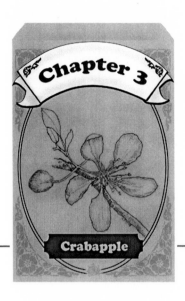

Chapter 3

Crabapple

Aeration: Loosen the Soil of Your Attitude

by Betsy

"I have learned from experience that the greater part of our happiness or misery depends on our dispositions and not on our circumstances."
~ Martha Washington

Aeration means loosening the soil to increase water saturation and make the soil more porous. Plant growth improves after aeration. Try aerating your attitude; stir things up by trying on different attitudes—cheerful, grumpy, stern, encouraging—and see how your world responds.

The importance of your attitude toward life

"You might as well laugh as cry," was my mother's mantra during her life. Instead of complaining about life's frustrations, we laughed about them. This philosophy gave my family strength to cope with difficulties with an attitude of humor and lightheartedness.

Kathleen and I attended our friend Mamie's sixtieth birthday party. It was a wonderful evening with music, stories, testimonials, and genuine joyfulness. Mamie was celebrating the influential women in her life who guided her, so all of the nearly one hundred fifty attendees were female. Mamie told us, "I've learned that the one thing we all have in common is the little girl in us. As long as she is still inside, we will never get old. That girl still has energy, dreams, and fun." Mamie's attitude radiates joyfulness and hope.

In his book *Authentic Happiness*, Dr. Martin Seligman gives us a method to rate our happiness.[1] Rate yourself on this scale making sure that the total is 100%. On average:

The percent of the time I feel happy is _____%.

The percent of time I feel unhappy is _____%.

The percent of the time I feel neutral is _____%.

Is the percent of the time you feel happy greater than the percent of the time you feel unhappy? What would you like for your averages to be?

Attitude vs. experiences

Why is attitude, the position with which you face the world, so important? Many people think that their experiences determine their attitude. ("She canceled lunch and it ruined my day.") Actually, the opposite is true—your attitude determines how you respond to your experiences. Some common questions include: Is having a positive or negative attitude genetic? Is it hard to change a person's attitude? The short answer to both is yes. You know people who seem to have a negative predisposition, and you no doubt have met others who typically seem very positive. The most common theory in the scientific community is that both nature (genetics) and nurture (environment) make significant contributions to attitude. According to psychologist Ed Diener, our capacity for happiness has a "baseline" measure, much like physical weight, with some people having a natural tendency to be cheerier than others.[2]

There is no one way to cope with the pains of life. People have different temperaments and cope with life in their unique way. Mary tells us that when her attitude is askew, she looks for something steady and finds that prayer is very grounding for her. She encourages people to "find your strength from a renewable source." In this chapter you will find additional methods for creating and strengthening an attitude that will benefit you in your abundant second half of life.

What was your attitude on life at age thirty or forty? Optimistic or pessimistic? What is it today? Is it different because of your life experiences? How do other people describe your attitude?

Dealing with discouragement

Whether you have a predominantly positive or negative attitude, there are times in life when all of us get discouraged, disappointed, or scared. Some days we feel lousy, so overwhelmed by the storm clouds that we can't see any lining—silver or any other color. Depending on your personality and the magnitude of the problem, it can be healthy to go with the bad feeling temporarily. Let yourself wallow in it. Give yourself permission to withdraw for a short period of time and don't try to be falsely cheerful. When you accept that you can cope in your own way and recover at your own pace, you will begin to feel better.

An effective technique is to give yourself a fixed amount of time for the misery. Choose a reasonable time when you will abandon the bad feeling and move forward. As we were writing the book, I moved from Pensacola, Florida, to Cary, North Carolina. Our moving company proved not to be the bargain we thought, as it took three weeks to get our household goods. One of my key strengths is fun and optimism; however, I became depressed and fearful that my household treasures were lost forever. I practiced positive self-talk: "It's only stuff. I can replace it." I still felt lousy. Kathleen gave me good advice that someone gave her years ago. "Think ahead three months from now. You'll know your way around your new city and have new friends." Her advice rang true and I soon came out of my doldrums.

Benefits of a positive attitude

There are many benefits of a positive attitude including coping with daily life better, being more optimistic about life, attaining goals more easily, and achieving success more rapidly. In addition, your ability to inspire and motivate yourself and others increases; you also experience fewer difficulties and have the power to surmount them due to your enhanced energy and greater inner strength. A positive outlook doesn't rid your life of problems, but it does help you deal with them more productively when they arise.

A twenty-year study of people fifty and older found that our attitude about aging affected how long we live. The study showed that people with a positive attitude about aging lived an average of 7.8 years longer than those who did not hold positive views about aging.[3]

Helpful ways to generate a more positive attitude

Decide. You can let your moods run your life, or you can override those swings by thinking and choosing your attitude. (Certainly, we're not talking about clinically depressed women who can benefit from medications.) After her ninety-four year old mother moved in with her, Mary's outlook plummeted. One day, she was asked to pick up eighty-eight year old Joan and take her to an activity. In contrast to Mary's mother, Joan's attitude was sunny. Mary told us the story: "Years ago, Joan's own elderly mother had been grumpy, so she decided *right then* not to grow old that way. She showed me what a decision can do. Now I think about my situation, 'It'll work. It'll be all right.' It's an intellectual thing, not emotional."

After decades of military moves, Maripaul's husband retired and her role as a military wife no longer existed. "I went through a long period of feeling depressed," she recalled. "Then I wrote myself a letter, asking, *What do I need to do? What's my attitude?*" She added, "I still have that letter. I typed it on the computer—in large font—and put it on the fridge where it's always visible. By writing it, I fessed up to myself that *I* am the only person who can get myself out of that dark place."

Exercise. If you do not currently exercise, start with small steps by creating a plan for regular exercise times. Invite a friend to join you. Both cardiovascular exercise (walking, running, swimming, and biking) and strength training (working with weights) are important. If it's financially feasible, hire a personal trainer for a while. Your attitude and abilities will improve by having a person who gives you his or her total attention for an hour, two or three days a week. Or join a dance class where you get a double dose of attitude enhancers—music and movement.

Laugh. As I mentioned early in the chapter, my family has a robust, if not unique, sense of humor. When my sister and I get together, we can still burst into hysterical laughter about stories of our childhood. To improve your outlook, laugh! A six-year-old child laughs three hundred times a day, but an adult laughs just forty-seven times a day.[4] Laughter is good for your soul and your body.

Laughter helps to remove stress by causing the release of natural painkillers in the body. When you laugh out loud, endorphins and adrenaline are released, which results in a natural high, making you feel good about yourself. It's also a good internal workout. A belly laugh exercises the diaphragm, contracts the abdominal muscles, works the shoulders, and even exercises the heart. Muscles relax after a good laugh.[5]

In our second half of life, we have the opportunity to establish new social networks and friends, but this can be stressful as well as rewarding. Laughter helps to connect us with others because it's contagious. You can bring more joy into the lives of others by laughing yourself. It also reduces your stress levels, both physically and psychologically.

Did you know that thirteen muscles are used for smiling and fifty muscles are used for frowning? You have to frown a quarter of a million times to make one wrinkle! In terms of exercise, you get the same benefits from laughing one hundred times a day as you can get from rowing for ten minutes.[6]

Mamie taught us about the girl in all of us. Set that little girl free. Try acting childlike (not childish). Chances are that whatever made you happy as a youngster still tickles your fancy. Eat chocolate ice cream, ride a bicycle, go to the zoo and chortle with the monkeys making faces at you, dig in the dirt, go to a parade, splash in a puddle instead of walking around it, make a sandcastle. Remember what gave you pleasure as a child and do it again.

Try these ways to increase laughter:
- Look for humorous moments every day.
- Watch comedies on television and at the movies.
- Read humorous books.
- Connect with a friend or relative with whom you can share your "funny memories."
- Look for the ridiculousness in frustrating situations.

Listen to music. Music is powerful, creating the mood for many settings. Think about the music you hear at parades. It's loud, fast-paced, rousing, and uplifting. The music played at sporting events inspires the athletes and engages the fans.

Music affects both the mind and body. The sound and rhythm have an effect on your cells and organs, and indirectly influence your emotions. In an experiment, when plants were exposed to classical music, their cells proliferated and produced larger, healthier plants. Music therapists and medical research show that the sound of music helps to manage pain, improve mood and mobility, reduce the need for pain relievers and sedatives associated with surgery, lower blood pressure, ease depression, and enhance concentration.[7]

Be adventurous by listening to a variety of radio stations. Attend a symphony performance. Expand your musical repertoire.

Keep a gratitude journal. Express gratitude often. Dr. Robert A. Emmons at the University of California, Davis, encourages people with depression to keep gratitude journals. He reports that people keeping such journals slept one half hour more per evening, woke up more refreshed, and exercised 33% more each week.[8] This journaling exercise helps you replace negative thoughts with positive ones. Every night as part of your bedtime routine, take a few minutes to record the things for which you are grateful that day.

Speak positively. Words have a powerful influence on people, so select your words and phrases carefully. "How was your day?" for example, is a phrase that most of us use in conversation. A typical response is, "Not too bad," which starts with a negative and literally means, "The day was crummy, but I survived." Consider using a more positive response such as, "I had a good day." "My day was productive." Or, "My day was busy but fulfilling."

Give compliments. It takes five positive interactions to undo the damage done with one negative comment.[9] What is your ratio of giving compliments versus criticizing? Do you tend to look for what is right and good, or what is wrong and bad, in yourself and in others? Giving sincere, deserved compliments creates a win-win for you and the person you compliment, uplifting both of your spirits.

To give meaningful compliments, follow these guidelines:
- Make sure the compliment is genuine. "You did a super job of organizing the fund-raiser. It raised a lot of money for the agency."

- Be specific with the compliment. "Your speech was great. It was timely, funny, informative, and your eye contact with the audience was excellent."
- Be timely. Compliment as soon as possible, not months after the event.
- Compliment in public; criticize in private.

Accept compliments graciously. For many women, it can be uncomfortable to receive compliments. I was golfing with a woman once who was much better than I was. When I praised her power and accuracy, she responded, "Wait until the back nine. I'll fall apart then." And of course since she expected to do poorly, she did. How do you usually respond to a compliment? When you're told that your outfit is lovely, do you reply with a "thank you" or do you say "this old thing?" When someone notices your ability to get things done, do you accept the praise, or decline it with, "Oh, anybody could have done it." A person with a positive attitude graciously gives and receives compliments. The best response to one is a simple, "Thank you."

Develop affirmations. Affirmations are statements of positive intentions, used as a technique to change negative self-talk into something positive. Affirmations are always stated in the first person ("I"), in the present tense (now), and are always positive. You want to convince your mind that *this has already happened.* Affirmations for women over fifty might include:

- I have value.
- I am making a useful contribution to my community.
- I possess a wealth of skills and experiences.
- I am a wise and wonderful woman.
- I am living my *Second Blooming.*

We'll explore affirmations more thoroughly in chapter 11. Keep this in mind as you prepare yourself for your own *Second Blooming*: events happen, but you choose the attitude with which you interpret them, and the behavior with which you will respond. This attitude adjustment can take some time. Mary, for example, said the final decision to leave her teaching career was pivotal. "After that, I decided God must have something else for me to do. Teaching was for a period of time, not forever." She had no control over her disease, only over how she chose to react to it.

Face your future with your most positive, productive outlook, because *you* determine how abundant your life will be. It will also prepare you to embrace and initiate the changes you want to make as discussed in the next chapter.

ACTIVITIES

Write down two ideas for increasing laughter in your life.

What three things did you enjoy as a child that you would like to experience again?

Listen to a variety of music. Write down what made you feel happy, sad, energized, calm, thoughtful, stressed, etc. Refer to this when you want to use music to affect your mood.

Give one sincere compliment to someone every day for a month. Note individuals' reactions to you as well as the impact on your own attitude.

Write down an affirmation that you will use for one month. Post it where you'll be reminded of it. What impact does it begin to have on your attitude after a week or two?

Lily

Lilies are the most stately
and varied of bulbous
plants. They have three
basic cultural requirements:
deep, loose, well-drained
soil; ample moisture year-
round (plants never
completely stop growing);
and coolness at roots with
some sun at tops where
flowers form. If clumps
become too crowded, dig
up, divide, and transplant
them in spring or fall. If
you're careful, you can lift
lily clumps at any time,
even in bloom.

— *The Southern Living
Garden Book, 275*

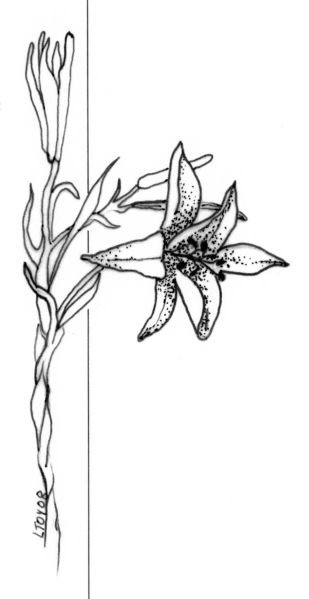

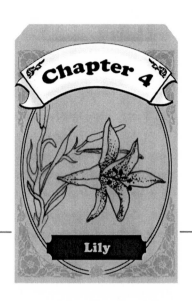

Chapter 4

Lily

Are You Root Bound? Embrace Change

by Kathleen

"We have to work our way up to saying, 'I'm not going to go backward. I'm not going to try to stay in the same place. That way lies self-torture and foolishness. I am going to have the courage to go forward.'" ~ Gail Sheehy

Are you root bound, held tightly in your life's pot, with roots clamoring for growth but circling uselessly at the bottom? Gardeners say to cut off the bottom third of such a plant, loosen the remaining roots, add new potting soil and the plant, then water thoroughly to energize new growth. I recently did such surgery on three plants. They behaved differently, but all were revitalized: the peace lily put out new shoots within the week; the hibiscus took longer, but bloomed more profusely than ever; the ficus immediately cheered up, putting out dozens of tiny, spring-green leaves. This process can be a metaphor for rejuvenating your life, too.

Like plants, women react differently to change. Some wilt, others perk up. "I have the boredom threshold of a three-year-old," says Betsy. "I'm always seeking change, so it's hard for me to see it as fearful." Shelby, too, said, "I love change. As a child, we moved many times. I like meeting interesting people. I adopted that philosophy about people. I don't find change stressful." Most women, including me, aren't nearly as open to change and the risks it involves as Betsy and Shelby are, but change happens, whether we seek it or not. After fifty, life is nothing if not an endless series of changes: our children marry, we become grandmothers, our parents grow old and die, knees and backs start to hurt, arthritis hobbles our fingers. And that's if everything happens in order. But add divorce, the death of a spouse or child, an unexpected move, a financial setback or major illness, and coping with change can easily seem daunting.

One of my major transitions came when my husband was diagnosed with cancer. Instantly our lives focused on learning everything we could about his options, meeting with specialists, then trying to determine the best way to proceed. Cancer and its challenges chose us, changing our lives and our outlook. Thankfully, he's fine now after surgery and radiation.

Other times, we can choose the changes we want to make. As much as I love my friends, family, and activities, I yearned to write in order to have a more lasting impact. So when Betsy asked, "Would you like to write a book with me?" I immediately said yes, and our lives were forever altered.

The connection between change and stress

Whether chosen or imposed on us, change is stressful. Why? Because every change is a story with a beginning, a middle, and an end. The problem is that you get "the end" first—the end of what's known, comfortable, and predictable. Then you have to deal with that very unsettling "middle" stage when you're not where you were, but it's not clear where you're going, either. You're like a trapeze artist who has let go of one rung midair, but hasn't yet caught the next rung to the other side. There is potential for danger here as you're suspended in air. For example, I'm sure you know someone who panicked after a divorce or her husband's death, and jumped too quickly into a bad relationship because she couldn't tolerate the feeling of being ungrounded. Understand, though, that a new beginning comes only after the work is done in that uncomfortable stage of uncertainty and suspension, which requires you to think, to analyze, to be aware of your choices, and to picture the likely consequences of those choices.

Women get stuck where they are, or jump too quickly into bad situations, because they're anxious or unsettled in that middle stage. Even a woman who can't stand her husband grieves deeply when he dies because her predictable world is shattered. With each ending, small or large, comes a loss, even when it's a desired change such as a son or daughter's marriage, or the arrival of grandchildren. There's a normal grieving process, ranging from minimal to intense, that accompanies each loss. As you contemplate changes you may want to make in your life, however, keep in mind that grief is usually more intense with events that are imposed on you and less so when you initiate or control the change.

Change involves risk

Risk makes many of us uneasy. For me, taking a risk raises feelings of fear and insecurity, but Betsy just gets excited. With practice, however, you can learn to put up with the tension as you make changes and work toward the goals you set. You'll learn to expect discomfort and disorientation before reaching your new orientation. Give yourself permission to take risks during the transition because they allow you to open yourself up to your many possibilities. As Mary said, "I view change as stressful, but I love the opportunities. I wouldn't have chosen some of the places we moved, but once the change happens, I'm capable of living in the moment. Now I would find it boring without change."

"Bad changes are harder to deal with," Beth acknowledged. "Is change risky? Of course." And Shirley admitted, "The older I get, I don't want to move anymore. I always do worry, but it always does seem to come out OK."

Maripaul found, "As a military wife, you know you're running in two or two and one-half year cycles. If things aren't great, you know you'll be leaving. But I chose to live each place as if I'd live there forever, and each place brought me new friends."

Emotionally, what can you expect?

If you know what to expect from the change process, you're less likely to be blindsided by it. Women often say they feel off balance, or out of control. They may feel varying levels of anxiety, frustration, and anger. Fear plays a huge role for many, too. Can I do this? Do I have my family's support? What if I fail? What if I made the wrong choice? And that comes with *choosing* change.

Sometimes you have little or no choice. My friend Nancy's husband, for example, was recently transferred unexpectedly to another state. She has moved several times and is an accomplished woman in many venues, but this time she thought they'd be staying in their home until he retired. After years of living in other countries, she finally had her family nearby. "I got really depressed," she confided. "A couple days, I couldn't even get out of bed. That's why you haven't seen me." She continued to feel confused, irritable, and insecure.

Nancy's behavior shows how inconsistent our reactions can be, depending on circumstances. "I've known nothing but change," shared Beth. "I've had to adapt. Sometimes I handle it gracefully, sometimes I don't." And, yes, your feelings may be mixed, with such emotions as anxiety and excitement co-existing.

Change affects your relationships

Be aware that when you initiate a change, your family and friends' lives are affected, too, because for every action, there is a reaction. When I went to work full time at our local United Way after two deadly hurricane seasons, my husband, who had just retired, picked up the household maintenance by shopping, cooking, and doing the laundry. This was a positive, supportive response, but when other men heard what he was doing, some said, "No way. I couldn't do that." In them, my change in work status would have provoked a different reaction: resistance or resentment.

Take time now to consider how you can prepare your family and friends for the changes you want to make. How is each person likely to react? What can you do to minimize any negative reaction and engage their support? How can you help them see the potential benefits to themselves as well as to yourself?

As women, we've often put our own desires on the back burner as we took care of our families and worked during the "responsible" years, so it can feel awkward to say, "At this point in my life, I want to _____." It may feel uncomfortable to acknowledge this mature stage of life, to identify your own needs and desires, and to start planning your *Second Blooming*.

Typical responses to change

How do people behave when facing change? There are several typical responses, which may vary depending on the situation. How many of these have you experienced over the years? Do you have a "favorite"?

- *Denial.* "I'm still young," or, "Change, what change?" Denial can be conscious or unconscious. Some employees I've had in seminars, for instance, refused to accept the reality of their company's announced closing, and were genuinely surprised at the last paycheck. Sometimes denial may be a conscious first step, temporarily buying time like Scarlett O'Hara's "I'll think about that tomorrow."

- *Good front.* You try to convince others you're ready for change, but you keep doing and thinking about things the same old way. Familiar routines make you feel safe and insulated.

- *Leave me out.* This is a "make all the changes you want, but leave me out" response. Nancy, for example, might have told her husband, "This is your transfer, not mine. I'm not going this time."

- *Go with the flow.* You make the absolute minimum adjustment necessary in your behavior. Nancy might have said, "OK, I'll go, but you'll have to arrange the move." You are lagging behind the change curve and the actions it demands of you.

- *Passive aggressive.* This is like a combination of "good front" and "leave me out." You invent schemes to undermine the real changes required of you. In Nancy's situation, she could have said, "Sure, I'll call the real estate office today," then conveniently "forget" to do it. Sabotage, whether mental or physical, is a real hazard.

- *Adaptation.* In this response, you deal with the reality of the situation as it arises, making necessary adjustments in your life. You ask yourself, for example, "Do I need to move? See a doctor? Talk to a counselor? Change jobs? Budget my money better?" Nancy had a good talk with herself to get to this point, and then successfully arranged the move. She chose to change her attitude, a step not necessary in past moves, which she had viewed with anticipation.

- *Anticipation.* You look ahead and see change coming, such as retiring or turning fifty with its "senior" designation, and plan accordingly. You're proactive, see the opportunities, and have begun asking, "What do I want for the rest of my life? What do I value? What skills do I have or need? What do I want to contribute?" You assess, plan, and take action, while looking forward to your *Second Blooming*.

Why should you seek change?

Change happens, ready or not. Every day, you're growing older. Don't you look in the mirror sometimes and wonder where those wrinkles came from? Or when your babies became adults? As the years continue to pass, your choices are to (1) embrace the opportunities open to you and initiate the changes you want, or (2) sit back and wait for things to happen *to* you and live with other people's decisions. Which do you prefer?

It helps to have some understanding of the big picture, too, so let's put life in a larger context. Carl Jung, Swiss psychiatrist and psychologist (1875–1961), was one of the first to recognize and divide our lives into four developmental stages: childhood, youth, middle life, and old age. Of middle life, he said, "If you desperately try to cling to your youth, you will fail in the process of self-realization."[1] With the acquisition of wisdom by old age, he believed, "people will not face death with fear but with the feeling of a 'job well done' and perhaps the hope for rebirth."[2]

Psychoanalyst Erik Erikson (1902–1994) expanded on Jung's view of the developmental stages with his classic 1950 book, *Childhood and Society*, in which he defined "The Eight Stages of Man." At our age, most of us find ourselves in Stage VII: Generativity vs. Stagnation. We need to know that our lives are being lived not just for ourselves, but also in relationship to humankind. In other words, a successful passage through this stage means we are concerned not just for our own egos and self-gratification, but also for others and the greater good. "Generativity is primarily the interest in establishing and guiding the next generation."[3]

Erikson's Stage VIII is Ego Integrity vs. Despair. This is when you reflect on your life and assess your efforts. Ego integrity, or being at peace with yourself, springs from your accomplishments in the earlier stages; despair comes with regret for a life not lived creatively, productively, abundantly.[4] You saw Jung and Erikson's influence on the Women's Growing Zones chart in chapter 2.

Costs of not changing

Choosing to do nothing or trying to maintain the status quo is a choice you can make, but be aware that there is a cost to you. Erikson called it Stagnation and Despair. Mary put it more bluntly: "Stagnation would make you 'swamp on down.' Staying the same isn't really neutral."

If you don't choose to think about, plan for, and live a life that matters from now on, be aware of the costs. You may:

___ forfeit your dreams;

___ cave in to your fears and insecurities;

___ miss your potential for an abundant life;

___ disappoint yourself;

___ waste your talents and gifts;

___ get stuck wondering "what if?"

___ suffer low self-esteem;

___ live an other-directed vs. self-directed life;

___ stagnate.

Check the one(s) which pose a cost to you if you fail to keep growing and never move into Zone 3.

Strategies for managing change productively

You already know there is a connection between exercise and a healthy body, but did you know there's also a correlation between "practicing" change and a mind that's flexible and ready for the future? Shirley, a nurse, said, "Change is good for your brain because it helps make new pathways."

Betsy says she's a "ready, fire, aim!" person. I'm slower, more analytical, hanging back until I gather information and get a sense of the big picture. We all have our usual ways of dealing with changes, but they can and must vary, depending on circumstances. Just as a single rose doesn't make a bouquet, neither does one approach to change make for a successful life.

Next are some of my favorite strategies for managing change. They've been tested in real life by real people: me, my family and friends, and people in seminars I've conducted.

1. *Train for change.* Practice being flexible. Take a different route home; sit on the opposite side at church (and enjoy people's startled reactions); eat a new kind of food; change the channel on your radio or television; buy a magazine you wouldn't normally read; put your watch on the other wrist. Try something new every week. What will it be this week?

_____

2. *Anticipate change.* Identify one change that's likely to happen in the next year of your life: a child will leave home, or will move back in? A marriage? Elderly parents will become sick or die? Leave your job? Take Social Security at sixty-two? Become eligible for Medicare at sixty-five? What do you need to know to manage this change, what skills must you develop, or what resources do you need to identify?

_____

3. *Build a "safety zone."* With a husband in the navy, I moved frequently. I don't do well with clutter, so stacks of boxes piled everywhere at the new house made me miserable by afternoon. I learned to choose the smallest, most manageable room, usually a half bath, make it as clean and nice as possible, then go there when my frustration level got high. I'd take a book or magazine, sit on top of the toilet seat, and read until I felt calm again. Other women have "mental" places to which they can escape, such as a vacation spot in the mountains or at the beach, a vision of a place they've traveled. What special place, physical or mental, makes you feel more tranquil? _____
Picture yourself there. Color in the images, remember the circumstances surrounding the event, and let yourself be completely engaged by them. Stay there until your breathing slows and you can sense your body letting go of tension.

4. *Accept your feelings.* Every change involves an ending and a loss. With the upcoming change you identified in #2, what do you see that you will lose? Might it be your home, a friend or family member, money, job, status, security? Now honor that loss by recognizing the feelings it generates in you. Are you: Resentful? Angry? Frustrated? Scared? Lonely? Irritable? Insecure? Excited? Bewildered? Thrilled? Confused?

Fearful? Grateful? Guilty? Relieved? Anxious? Sad? You get the idea. Be specific. _____ Now, own the feelings, remembering that feelings aren't good or bad, they just exist. They do give you information, however, for the choices of behavior you can then make.

5. *Set a time boundary.* When we moved to Japan, I was immediately hospitalized with pneumonia. The next day, my husband had to fly out to meet the ship at sea; fortunately, a dear friend was there who kept our nine-year-old son, but I just wanted to go home to my mother. A navy wife I'd never met visited me at the hospital and advised, "I know you're miserable now, but give it three months. By then, you'll be well, be able to count yen, find your way off base, and take the train to Tokyo." I didn't believe her, but it all came true, just as she predicted, because my unconscious mind worked to meet that deadline. I passed on this strategy to Betsy when she recently moved to North Carolina, and it worked for her, too. How many days, weeks, or months is it reasonable to expect yourself to adapt to your change? _____ Write it on the calendar.

6. *Talk with others.* No, this isn't a "pity party" or a time to gripe and complain. Instead, choose people who can be useful sounding boards for you, who will listen thoughtfully and may have practical suggestions. If they have been successful in handling similar situations, ask how they did it, what their management techniques were. The more we share productively with each other, the more we all grow in our life skills. What two people do you know who are most likely to be helpful in making your change?_____

7. *Take care of yourself.* Coping with change adds stress to your life, so it's especially important to exercise, eat good food, and get enough sleep. Under pressure, though, you may be tempted to eat fast food, cheat on exercise, or cut back on sleep. Which of those three areas are you most likely to sacrifice when you're stressed? What do you plan to do to keep yourself healthy throughout the change process?

_____

8. *Understand the "why."* Ask questions so you are armed with facts instead of rumors or misconceptions. What's behind this change? For example, is the company being downsized? Will your job be eliminated in the merger? Why is your mother's health deteriorating so quickly? Realize, too, that sometimes there can be no answer. Some events just strike at random, such as when your only son develops Crohn's disease, your husband is diagnosed with cancer, or your niece dies in a car crash. In those situations, your only productive choice is to keep living, to try to make some lasting good come out of the tragedy. But if you *can* ask what's behind the change, do so. What's precipitating your change?

_____

9. *Face reality.* Accept your situation. Denial doesn't get you anywhere, and neither does wishful thinking. Some examples of statements facing reality could include:
   • My job will be eliminated within the year.
   • My husband is being transferred to another state.
   • Mom has Alzheimer's.
   • I just turned fifty and received an application for membership from AARP.
   Only when you acknowledge reality can you begin to prepare for your future. What is one statement of your reality?

_____

10. *Identify your Circle of Influence.* In his book *The Seven Habits of Highly Effective People*, Stephen R. Covey describes a large "circle of concern," and within it, a smaller "circle of influence."[5] You have many issues that concern you, but you cannot influence all of them, so spend your time—your life—on those issues that you can affect. For example, you can't stop a bank merger or your mother's Alzheimer's, but you *can* decide whether or not to stay with the bank, or what treatment options to pursue for mom. Is there any part of your change that is outside your circle of influence? _____Don't waste your time worrying about it. What part of the change *can* you influence or control? _____ In many ways,

Covey's circles of concern and influence are a picture of the familiar Serenity Prayer: Grant me the serenity to accept the things I cannot change, the courage to change the things I can, and the wisdom to know the difference.

11. *List the obstacles.* Many things can get in the way of successfully making your change. They might include a negative attitude, an unwillingness to take the risk, wishful thinking, a lack of skills or education, insufficient information, or no experience. What obstacles do you see standing between you and making this change success-fully? _____ (Chapter 5 may also help you with this.)

12. *Look for opportunities.* Every change, desired or not, holds within it the potential for opportunity. For instance, the bank merger may lead to a promotion. A nursing home may mean better health care for your mother and peace of mind for you. Your husband's transfer may open a whole new culture for you to explore. What possible opportunities might your change offer? Be creative and list several, no matter how "wild" they may seem to you now.

Once you're aware of the benefits that may come with change, you'll find yourself more open to, and engaged in, the process.

Know what not to change

It's essential to hold on to the essence of who you are, whatever your age. "Some things you don't want to change, like values," said Shelby. "Stay true to that one thing that's really important."

Mary added, "Yes, things that anchor your roots."

For Beth, "I like people who hang onto those bedrock things. I respect people who are consistent."

Their message? As you seek change, be true to yourself and your core values. The emphasis on them may shift, but they are integral to your authentic self.

Looking ahead

Embrace change. Yes, it involves risk, which may make you uneasy, but the potential rewards of joy and soul-filling abundance are worth it. You may not know yet what changes you want to make in your life, and that's OK. In this chapter, you've primed yourself by increasing your knowledge and practicing a variety of change strategies so you'll be ready when you *do* have a vision.

Between you and that vision, however, are some obstacles or "weeds," which could stunt your *Second Blooming*. The next chapter will help you identify them, with tips for minimizing their impact.

ACTIVITIES

What's your most frequent response to change (e.g., passive-aggressive)? Pick a different response and try using it for two weeks. Assess how it worked for you.

Think about a change in the past that didn't go well. Knowing what you do now, is there another strategy you could have used? How might the outcome have been different?

You identified a change that will probably happen to you soon. What three strategies are most likely to help you adapt to this change?

ADDITIONAL RESOURCE

Who Moved My Cheese? by Spencer Johnson, M.D.

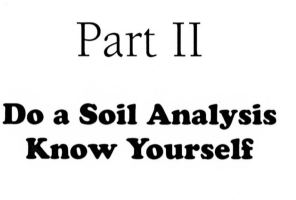

Part II

Do a Soil Analysis
Know Yourself

Kudzu

Kudzu is known as "The Vine That Ate the South." It has covered millions of acres since it was introduced in 1876. It smothers arbors, telephone poles, houses, and fields—and any plant in its path—at the rate of up to one foot per day, thriving under almost any condition. It's too invasive for garden use unless you're hiding from the government and need something to cover your tracks.

— *The Southern Living Garden Book, 345*

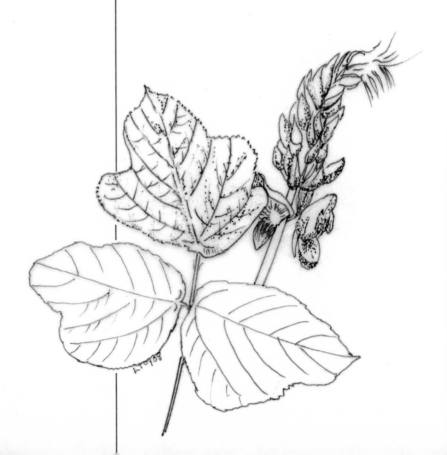

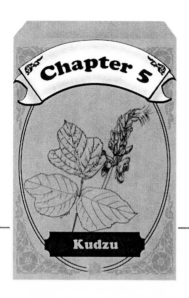

Chapter 5

Kudzu

Weeds: Pull Them to Improve Your Life Garden's Yield

by Kathleen

"Out, damned spot! Out, I say!"
~ Shakespeare's Lady Macbeth

In this chapter, we'll identify a number of common behaviors, which, like kudzu, can stifle your growth by smothering your energy and creativity. Start clearing them from your life or risk remaining stuck and unfulfilled. Think of them as weeds that need to be pulled in preparation for your spring planting.

Usually, Betsy and I select pieces of the conversations we have with the women, but for this chapter, the whole exchange seemed so relevant that we want to share it in its entirety. As you'll see, we all deal with similar issues in our lives. Read, too, with a mind for what interferes with your life.

Kathleen: Where do these "weeds" or self-destructive behaviors— like perfectionism, addictions, or excessive debt—come from?

Beth: They stem from a lack of self-awareness or self-examination.

Mary:	From fear.
Kathleen:	What does it cost women to continue these behaviors?
Beth:	They surrender creativity for safety and stability. Women are aware of what they're doing. For instance, I think every addict knows that she's addicted.
Mary:	We sabotage ourselves by misuse of time, too. My husband and I are being sabotaged by watching too much television.
Kathleen:	I often do the less important stuff on my to-do list just so I can see more things checked off.
Mary:	Me, too. The big things don't get done and keep being transferred to the next to-do list. Like cleaning out my files. But I got smart last month. I took the box in the car when we were traveling. I was trapped and had to clean it out.
Kathleen:	How do you convince yourself that now's the time to do something, to make a change?
Beth:	Be honest with yourself. And in your book, *show* women, because some people don't know how to stop or change their behavior.
Mary:	You need to be able to weigh your potential gains and losses. Ask yourself: how badly do I want what I don't have now?
Beth:	Don't excuse yourself too easily, but do expect some derailing as you try to change. Also, if you're staying in an abusive or unsupportive marriage, ask yourself why. What's keeping you there?

Mary: Or why you're not working to change the relationship to meet *your* needs, too.

Beth: There's a risk here. Like, if you think about leaving a bad marriage, are you willing to risk being poor? And sometimes your attitude and expectations of marriage are off-kilter. An older marriage is different than a younger one.

Mary: So many people don't know what to realistically expect from a marriage.

Kathleen: For some women, there's physical or emotional abuse…

Mary: …anger and resentment…

Beth: …or blame, like blaming your parents for what they did or didn't do in raising you.

Kathleen: Maybe we can "reframe" that blame, and chalk it up to misunderstanding or a lack of skill or maturity in our parents or whomever.

Mary: Look at whatever issues you're dragging forward with you. Check them off. Just decide your parents did the best they could. Then you can take ownership of your life and ask: what are my blessings? What can I do *now* instead of wasting my energy on the past?

Beth: Also ask yourself why you're hanging on to this blame. What's the payoff? What's it doing for you?

Mary: Oh, yes: Righteous anger. I heard somewhere that anger and resentment are like drinking a little poison every day and expecting the *other* person to get sick.

Kathleen:	Are there other behaviors that are self-destructive?
Beth:	Sure. When faced with a sensitive issue, be aware of the dynamics. I was trying to set up a family photo recently. One of my brothers was blinded by anger and didn't want to include another brother. I felt rattled, and could easily been de-railed by buying into his anger. If I had acquiesced, it would have broken my heart! There are traps in my family that I don't even know are there.
Kathleen:	And if you gave in, you'd be giving away your integrity, your self.
Mary:	Integrity is *so* important. It goes back to knowing and trusting yourself.
Kathleen:	So you need to surround yourself with people who won't derail you.
Betsy:	At this point in life, many of our relationships have changed. For example, our kids are grown. Also, when I retired from my job, I found out which relationships were work-related and which were real friendships. And both were OK.
Kathleen:	I heard once that we have friends for a reason, a season, or a lifetime. It can be harmful to try to force a relationship into something it wasn't meant to be.
Mary:	Everybody has issues, but we need to cut people some slack. Like, after she moved here, my mom didn't hear from a friend for six years. But when she did, she complained. I just said, "Mom, be glad. Let it go."
Beth:	Forgiveness is an excellent tool for "letting it go," but I didn't know *how* to forgive. It seems easy, straightforward, but it's not.

Kathleen: I hate that saying, "forgive and forget." You can't really forget, but you can forgive. It's hard work, but it frees *you*. You can choose to stop whatever happened from running and ruining your life.

Mary: I heard at church that if you do what you've always done, you'll be what you've always been.

Betsy: Yes, the definition of insanity is doing the same thing again and again, but expecting a different result.

Mary: So why is changing our behavior so hard?

Betsy: There's comfort in routines and predictability.

Kathleen: Why should women stop their self-destructive behaviors, whatever they are?

Beth: Because they hurt!

Mary: Realize what you *could* be doing with your life if you got rid of them.

Identifying your weeds

Now it's time for you to decide if you have any "weeds" you want to pull in preparation for your *Second Blooming*. First, choose the issues from the list on the next page (preferably no more than three) that cause you the most trouble by asking yourself: does this interfere with my well-being and relationships? Does it keep me from living my life as fully as I want?

Inventory of "weeds" or behaviors that inhibit personal growth

You can also print this inventory from:

www.secondbloomingforwomen.com

ISSUE:

___ Abuse (physical, emotional, verbal)

___ Addictions (gambling, alcohol, legal or illegal drugs, food, smoking)

___ Anger

___ Blame

___ Debt

___ Guilt, regret

___ Passivity or aggressiveness

___ Perfectionism

___ Procrastination

___ Stress

___ Time

___ Worry, anxiety

___ Other _____ (You know best what's holding you back.)

If you didn't check any issues, you may proceed to chapter 6. If you checked one or more, keep reading.

Prepare to take action on your issue(s)

Commit to taking action, which has several immediate rewards: your attitude will likely improve (because you'll be doing what you know you need to); you will release physical and mental energy that you've been expending on negative activities; and you will begin to glimpse a different future for yourself.

Common advice over the years has been to tackle one problem at a time. Stop smoking first, for example, and then cut down on watching television. However, a recent medical study covered in *AARP The Magazine* challenged that idea. Doctors "asked patients to quit smoking, reduce their salt intake, and walk an extra 1500 steps a day. The results? Those who were asked to change all their bad habits at once (rather than one habit at a time) tended to fare better."[1]

If you revert to your old behavior out of habit, forgive yourself and try again. That same issue of *AARP* reported, "40% of resolution makers succeed on the first try; 17% try six or more times before they succeed."[2] Be persistent.

Now you're ready to proceed. Go to the pages covering the issues you selected (they're in alphabetical order) where you'll find background information, tips, and additional resources. Decide what action you'll take, writing it on notes posted where you'll constantly be reminded (e.g., on the front of the computer). Use this different and conscious choice of behavior as situations arise. If you're keeping a journal, jot down the circumstances, how you probably would have reacted in the past, and how this new behavior worked out. Be patient with yourself, remembering that change is a process, not a one-time event. Once you've read about the issues you checked, you may skip to the last paragraph of this chapter.

Keep in mind, please, that this is not a therapy book; we're coaching, not counseling. If you find you need more than we offer here, start by contacting some of the additional resources given at the end of each section, or seek professional help.

> *Reach deep inside*
> *Pull hard on fear*
> *Shake loose complacency*
> *Strip away hurt*
> *Be gone*
> *Throw them out!*
> *~ Shelby Miller*

Abuse (physical, emotional)

"One-third to one-half of adult women has been abused by their spouse or significant other."[3] Shocking? Yes. And it occurs at all socioeconomic levels. You do not deserve to be hit or abused, and you do not cause it. The batterer is responsible for his abusive behavior, using violence as an ineffective way of problem-solving or exerting power.

What kinds of abuse are there? Physical (slapping, hitting, burning); sexual (when, where, and how he wants it without regard for your feelings); verbal (yelling, rage, threats, and intimidation); psychological and emotional (e.g., you're useless, ugly). Abusers tend to blot out feelings other than anger, trying very hard to be their vision of "manly." In general, they don't know how to handle frustration, anger, or conflict.

Both the victim and the abuser feel trapped because: they don't see a way out; there's a basic lack of protection; they feel fear and shame, and isolated in their predicament. Yet hope and love are not necessarily extinguished, with caring and affection often still existing. Although more often it is the male who is the batterer, there are also women who resort to violence. Abuse is not acceptable for either sex.

Being in an abusive relationship is an unhealthy way to live. If this is your situation, you have three choices:

1. Leave him. Have a plan and be careful.
2. Choose to stay and hope he will change; enlist outside help.
3. Stay, but give up hope that he'll change; endure the abuse. (If this is your choice, your ability to live a *Second Blooming* is severely limited.)

If you've been in this situation, you probably know that violence tends to escalate over time. As we mentioned, this is not a therapy book, and abuse can't be addressed in a paragraph. However, we suggest that you be prepared ahead of time. Some things you can do:

• Have a safe place to escape.
• Identify supportive people. (Abusers usually isolate the abused from friends and family, so this may take some effort.)
• Believe in your right to a violence-free life.
• Have some emergency money.

TIPS:
• *Admit your problem and seek help, such as a counselor. Go alone if he won't go with you.*
• *Look up your local women's shelter (see Crisis Intervention Services or Social and Human Service Organizations in the phone book, or call your local United Way) and keep the number(s) handy.*

Addictions

There are numerous addictions (gambling, alcohol, legal or illegal drugs, food, smoking) but at their heart, they all have a similar basis:

they're a way for us to avoid living our lives head-on. Addictions involve "stuffing" the normal emotions of life. When women lack the personal resources or skills to face their lives and situations squarely, they may take refuge in various addictions. Anne Wilson Schaef says the "function of an addiction is to put a buffer between ourselves and our awareness of our feelings. An addiction serves to numb us so that we are out of touch with what we know and what we feel."[4]

It's not just emotional pain that you submerge with your addiction. I have a dear friend, Brenda, of many decades. Yes, we often had wine together, but I had no idea that she'd stay up after her husband went to bed, drinking from bottles she'd hidden around the house. One night she fell down a flight of stairs, scaring herself and her husband who dashed downstairs to check on the noise. Embarrassed and shocked into action, she started attending Alcoholics Anonymous and quit drinking. The most astonishing thing was yet to come. I knew she had begun taking some painting classes and expected a beginner's efforts, but when she opened her car trunk after class one day, I was dumbstruck at the exquisite landscape. "You did this?" I marveled.

"Yes," she said.

I had to ask, "Where did this talent come from and where has it been hiding all these years?"

She answered, "I guess it was covered up by the alcohol. I had no idea I could paint. It's a gift." She was clearly as surprised as I was.

Putting it bluntly, you need to feel the emotional pain that you've tried so hard to mask with your addiction of choice. Acknowledge your addiction, and then decide whether you want to keep it, or give yourself permission to let it go and move in another direction. As with Brenda, it absorbs your time, energy, and creativity, keeping you from even a hint of a *Second Blooming*. You have a real choice: a life stunted by addiction, or a life lived fully with eyes and heart wide open to possibilities.

When you're tempted by your addiction and are about to give in to it, pause and ask yourself:
- What feelings am I trying to cover up?
- What do I gain by continuing this addiction?
- What does it cost me?
- How might my life be different if I gave it up? What are the potential benefits?

TIP:
If you have an addiction, fill in the blanks:
I'm addicted to

_____.

This addiction started when I

_____.

I keep hanging onto my addiction because

_____.

If I gave it up, I would be able to

_____.

As a first step in conquering my addiction, I will

_____.

RESOURCES:
Gamblers Anonymous (GA)	*www.gamblersanonymous.org*
Alcoholics Anonymous (AA)	*www.aa.org*
Narcotics Anonymous (NA)	*www.na.org*
Overeaters Anonymous (OA)	*www.oa.org*

Your physician or local hospital, counselor, or other professional

Anger

In 1993, I led a daylong seminar for women who ranged in age from seventeen to eighty. By far, the most revealing session was the one on anger. The oldest essentially said, "I don't get angry, it's not ladylike." Women like me in their forties and fifties said, "I was brought up that way, too, but now I admit that I do get angry." We were straddling the fence between generations, brought up one way, but retraining ourselves and bringing up our daughters differently. The teenage girls simply said, "Do I feel anger? Sure. What's the problem?"

Many of us over fifty still find anger unsettling, but it's just an emotion, a feeling, and a perfectly normal one. Everyone experiences anger; it's neither right nor wrong, it just is. On the plus side, anger alerts you that something is wrong; it energizes you to defend yourself or someone else, and helps give you the courage to take action.

Your behavior, however, the action you take, is a choice, and some choices of behavior work better than others. You can:

- *Stuff it!* With this, you "swallow" your anger, denying your feeling, pretending it doesn't exist. The potential cost for this choice? You feel helpless, your self-esteem suffers, and the problem that generated the anger doesn't get solved. This is a "You win, I lose" approach.

- *Escalate it!* This includes name-calling, profanity, yelling, violence, abuse, or simply steamrolling over the other person. You may "win" in the short term, but the cost is high because others will resent you, and you'll become isolated as they stay out of your aim. Escalation never generates a good outcome; instead, the problem gets worse. It's an "I win, you lose" approach.

- *Direct it!* You're assertive, expressing yourself in a way that might lead to a solution. This approach respects both you and the other person, leaving your self-esteem intact. It's an "I win-you win" approach toward solving the problem instead of letting it fester or escalate.

TIPS:
- *Admit when you're feeling angry.*
- *Take a deep breath and count to ten (or a hundred…or take a thirty-minute walk) to cool down.*
- *Ask yourself: on a scale of 1 to 10, how angry am I? To help you decide, pick a number or circle the word that most closely describes how you feel:*

bugged	*angry*	*enraged*
irritated	*ticked off*	*furious*
annoyed	*mad*	*explosive*
bothered	*agitated*	*murderous*
(1 to 3)	*(4 – 7)*	*(8 – 10)*

Column 1 (1-3) is low-level anger; consider a minor response or just let it go.
Column 2 (4-7) is mid-level anger; you do need to take appropriate action.
Column 3 (8-10) is major anger, so be careful not to let your emotions run away from you. Defuse your emotions before taking action.

- *Don't try to prove you are right or morally superior; instead, clarify the problem.*
- *Ask yourself: no matter how it happened, what can I do about the situation now?*
- *Stay task-oriented; focus on the issue and solving the problem.*

Blame

"What do women say when they're blaming other people or circumstances instead of taking responsibility for their own lives?" Betsy and I asked the women. They were quick with examples:

"You shouldn't have left that statue where Timmy could knock it down."

"It's my boss' fault."

"My husband won't let me do that."

"I can't help it. I was raised in an abusive home."

"I'll never get a job that pays well because my parents didn't encourage me to go to college."

There must be a benefit for placing blame outside ourselves, but what is it? Mary felt, "It's self-justification for not doing something." Beth added, "It shifts responsibility away from yourself." The end result is that your life seems out of your control. You become a victim.

Making excuses for yourself by blaming others is a sign that you've given up ownership of your life, that you've empowered other people. When you're thirteen, telling your friends, "My parents won't let me do that" is age-appropriate. But when you're a woman over fifty? It's time to claim your life, not indulge in blame. As a friend said, "Self-responsibility is the highest form of maturity."

On the news, I heard an example of blame taken to the extreme. A woman had gambled until she lost her job, her home, and nearly a million dollars. Incredibly, she was suing six casinos for twenty million dollars because they should have seen that she had a problem and stopped her. In her mind, it was the casinos' fault.

There's an interesting twist to blame, too, as Mary has seen. "This happens a lot with my mother. One small infraction and *everything* is wrong. Yesterday, she made one small spill, then blamed herself for everything: 'I'm such a messy person. I'm always spilling something. I'm such a burden to you.'" Rather than projecting blame on others, Mary's mother took too much upon herself, far past the simple "I'm sorry" that the situation warranted.

TIPS:
Repeat to yourself, "I am not a victim. I am responsible for my own life."
Ask, "What role did I play in this situation?" and, "What can I learn from it?"
If you take too much responsibility, determine: on a scale of 1-10, this situation is worth a ____.

Debt

Debt compromises your future. If you want to live your dreams, you must stop deficit spending. Debt is a stressor, making you vulnerable not just financially, but physically and emotionally, as well.

"Why change now?" you may wonder. "I've been OK so far." Here are some facts from Sandra Block's column "Your Money" in *USA Today*: First, the average sixty-two-year- old woman will live 25.5 more years, and the average sixty-two-year-old man another 21.9 years. Second, more than 40% of elderly women depend on Social Security for more than 90% of their income, compared with 28% of elderly men. Social Security was designed as a safety net, not a retirement program. Third, because women live longer than men and tend to be younger than their husbands, they can expect several years of widowhood and major reductions in their standard of living. Fourth, more than 20% of unmarried women over 65 are poor.[5]

There are only two ways to increase your income: generate more, or spend less. Since we live in a consumer-driven economy, it will take a change of attitude and behavior to ignore advertisements imploring you to "buy this because you deserve it."

Some ways you can begin to reduce debt:
- Pay off credit card debt; put nothing more on your cards.
- Use cash rather than credit for major purchases so you'll save interest charges.
- Draft a budget, and stick to it; write down every cent you spend daily.

- Don't even open the next solicitation for a credit card; just take the scissors to it and toss out the pieces.

TIPS:
- *Before making a purchase, ask yourself, "Is this a <u>want</u> or a <u>need</u>?"*
- *If it's a want, decide whether you prefer short-term pleasure or long-term security.*
- *Wait one day before making the purchase.*
- *Use a reputable credit counseling agency to educate yourself and get back on track.*

RESOURCES

National Foundation for Credit Counseling, www.nfcc.org

Association of Independent Consumer Credit Counseling Agencies www.aiccca.org

Guilt, regret

Guilt and regret are like two flowers on a single stem—intimately related, yet each with a distinct bloom. Regret looks backward, and you feel sorrow or remorse for something you did or didn't do. You made a decision, chose a course of action, and it didn't turn out well. "I *could* have handled it differently," you think. Regret is a form of feedback to you if you pay attention to its signal, allowing you to learn from your mistakes and use your experiences to be smarter in the future.

When you find yourself thinking, "I *should* have handled it differently," you're experiencing guilt. You feel remorse for something you did or didn't do, and are distressed because you violated your personal values or beliefs.

On the good side, regret and guilt indicate you have a conscience, so they can be helpful to you if you heed their warnings. On the down side, they can take over like kudzu, stifling your potential for growth. It can be helpful to remember that you aren't the same person who made that mistake or violated your values because ideally you've changed and evolved into a new and better person since the incident. You don't have to stay stuck in regret and guilt. Instead, take that mental energy and put it to better use. Make something good come out of your distress.

TIPS:

- *Can you make amends by apologizing or setting things right? Be big enough to do so, if possible. Also, what lesson did you learn?*

- *Try redirecting negative energy into something related and positive you can do now. What are your options?*

- *Write a letter to the person, whether dead or alive, sharing your feelings. Mailing it is optional.*

RESOURCE

"Woulda, Coulda, Shoulda" by David Dudley. *AARP The Magazine.*

Passive or aggressive behavior

Do you know women who seem to get what they want and need in life without alienating others? They're undoubtedly assertive. What's important for you to know is that being assertive is a skill, which can be learned with some basic instruction and practice, although it does come easier to some women than others. The goal? To develop self-confidence and an alternative to powerlessness and manipulation by others.

You may recall the book *I'm OK—You're OK* by Thomas A. Harris, M.D. published in 1969. It can help you understand the definitions for the three basic styles of interacting with others:

1. Passive. This orientation is "You're OK, I'm not." You're apologetic; put others' wants and needs before your own, perhaps thinking you're being polite; are inhibited; allow others to make decisions for you; often feel hurt, anxious, and frustrated (but you stuff these feelings inside); and you're unlikely to achieve your desired goals. You're a doormat.

   - Advantages? You don't have to take responsibility for making decisions; you minimize your risk of taking a stand on issues; you avoid overt conflict.

- Disadvantages? You're likely to experience a sense of impotence; lower self-esteem; have to live with others' decisions; problems aren't solved.

2. Aggressive. This is an "I'm OK, you're not" outlook. You consider your personal needs while dismissing others' needs and wants; you achieve your desired goals even if it hurts or humiliates others; you project an "It's my way or the highway" attitude. You're brash, rude, obnoxious, and thoughtless.
   - Advantages? Other people give in to your demands; you have a sense of power and control; you "win" in the short run.
   - Disadvantages? You create resentment, humiliation, and guilt in your relationships; you alienate others, making your life lonely; aggression may lead to violence or emotional abuse; you're unable to get your wants or needs met in the long run.

3. Assertive. This says, "I'm OK, you're OK." You value your own needs but take others' needs into account, too; you make your own choices and decisions; you maintain an attitude of mutual respect; you state your thoughts and feelings honestly; you're willing to problem-solve and compromise. Being assertive allows you to:
   - ask for what you want;
   - not feel guilty;
   - not be pushed around by others;
   - respect people's individuality;
   - be flexible;
   - admit mistakes;
   - take responsibility;
   - let others know of your expectations;
   - state your views clearly;
   - have healthy relationships.

Sounds good, doesn't it?

Actually, you are capable of all three of these styles, depending on the situation. If it's just not worth a fuss, you may decide to be passive, to let the other person have his or her own way. If it's a dangerous situation, you may aggressively take charge, yelling orders as needed. One caveat: watch out for the evil combination, "passive-aggressive." It's the classic "Yes, of course; I'll do that right away" while thinking "Over my dead body." It's saying one thing but doing another—a wimpy way of being aggressive.

Remember: It is within your power to become more assertive.

TIPS:
Use "I" when talking about yourself (I want…I see…I need…).
Practice the three-step method: When you…I feel…I want…
(Example: "When you say I'm too old to go to school, I feel put down and diminished. I want you to support me in taking this class.")

Perfectionism

There's a strong connection between perfectionism, procrastination, and low self-esteem. Your negative self-talk (that chatter inside your head) might go something like this: "This project has to be perfect or people will think poorly of me, that I'm dumb. But I don't know enough yet, so I'd better read and study more before I get started." Or as Mary put it, "If I can't do it just right, I don't do it at all, so the piles of papers are still on my kitchen table." You are not perfect and never will be, but so what? You're a wonderful, competent person. We are, after all, human *beings*, actively stretching, learning, growing, and changing. Striving for excellence rather than perfection is liberating, and you're likely to accomplish more with less stress.

TIP:
Say and think, "I will strive for excellence" and "I will do my best" instead of "It has to be perfect."

Procrastination

What causes women to put things off? One factor is a fear of failure; another is feeling inadequate for the task. Some typical thoughts might be: "I'm not smart enough. I don't know how to do this. What if I mess up? What if I don't like the result? What if I fail?" Or you may feel overwhelmed, unable to find a starting place.

Fear of change may be another contributor. After reading chapter 4, you know a lot about this one. Probably the biggest cause of procrastination is perfectionism, or wanting the outcome to be picture-perfect, flawless. If perfection is unattainable, why start?

TIPS:

- *Divide the task into smaller parts. Betsy and I, for example, wrote this book one chapter at a time. Have a mental picture of the whole task, but focus on completing one step at a time.*
- *Tell someone what you want to accomplish so he or she can help hold you accountable. Betsy and I had so many friends asking, "How's the book coming? When can I buy it?" that we couldn't possibly have quit.*
- *Schedule your next step. For example: "I'll finish the first draft of chapter 5 by the end of this month." Write it on your calendar.*
- *Quit being passive, using such excuses as, "There isn't enough time," or, "It isn't getting done." Be honest. Use the active, responsible voice: "I am putting it off."*
- *Face an unpleasant task squarely. This is hard! But putting it off increases your stress and anxiety as it looms out there, waiting for you to take action, so do it first.*
- *Reward yourself on completion of the project or major steps of it.*

Stress

As you know, there's good stress and bad stress. The good stuff gets you up and moving in the morning, and is challenging, energizing, and motivating. But even desired events, like a child's marriage or choosing a new direction in life, can cause stress. And, yes, you can feel both excited and anxious at the same time.

Bad stress—like layoffs, financial losses, injury or death, earthquakes or floods—affects us physically, mentally, emotionally, and spiritually. It can cause a wide variety of symptoms, such as an upset stomach, headache, back pain, and an inability to think clearly.

The biggest source of stress, and potentially the biggest stress reducer, isn't external, but rather your perception of the situation. You can consciously and deliberately choose how you'll react to a situation. Be alert to negative choices of behavior, which include:

- doing nothing, hoping it will just go away (Caution: As a woman in one of my seminars said, "You can sweep your problem under the rug, but you'll keep tripping over the bump it makes.");
- seeking fast, temporary relief through drugs, alcohol, food, etc.;
- taking it out on others through physical, verbal, or emotional abuse.

It's not hard to see how counterproductive these strategies are, but what does work?

I've done hundreds of stress management seminars, lasting from one to eight hours, covering a wide variety of useful strategies, but the single most useful one, elegant in its simplicity, comes from my husband. As a navy fighter pilot, Flack flew combat missions over Vietnam. Many of his friends were being shot down, killed, or captured. In the middle of the war, he flew home on R & R (rest and recreation) for two weeks. In the grocery store, his brother "went ballistic" over the perceived high price of tomatoes, while Flack thought silently, *"Big deal!"* And so his "Big Deal" theory was born. On a scale of one to ten, having someone trying to kill you is a ten, he decided, and everything else is less than that.

To illustrate further, have you ever had surgery and had the nurse ask, "On a scale of one to ten, how bad is the pain?" You assessed and numbered your pain, and she gave an appropriate medical response to reduce it. The Big Deal theory works the same way, except that it's mental or emotional pain. You don't need morphine for a hangnail, nor do you need to have a major reaction to a minor issue.

TIPS:
- *When faced with a stressful situation, stop, take a deep breath, and ask yourself, "On a scale of one to ten, how big a deal is this to me?"*
- *Then choose an appropriate level of response.*

Time management

Do you too often find the day gone without any sense of satisfaction or accomplishment? Rich or poor, we all live in the same framework of twenty-four hours a day, seven days a week, or "24/7" as it's come to be known. But what great differences there are in how much individuals accomplish. Bad decisions lead to frustration, lower self-esteem, and increased stress. And people who don't have good time management skills are usually the ones who "don't have time" to learn how to improve them.

I believe there's an additional factor for women because we've often spent years organizing our lives around others' needs: the boss wants the report tomorrow; son's soccer practice Tuesday and Thursday; daughter's piano lesson Wednesday; husband's office party Friday, etc. We've been responders, filling our calendars with everyone else's required activities, sometimes forgetting our own needs. After fifty, your calendar may become free of many external obligations, but you might not be accustomed to choosing and scheduling activities for yourself. It's time to make yourself a priority.

Recognize, too, the difference between efficiency and effectiveness: being efficient means doing the job right, but being effective means *doing the right job*. You can be efficient all day long but accomplish nothing of value. When you write down your "to do" list, it shouldn't be more than ten items. Resist the temptation to do the easy ones first so you can have several items checked off (efficient). Also, the 80/20 rule, or the Pareto principle, "means that in anything, a few (20 percent) are vital and many (80 percent) are trivial."[6] Applied to time management, then, 20% of your activities can produce 80% of desired results *if* you do the one or two most *important* items on your list (effective).

TIPS: ask yourself…
- *Is this activity helping me reach my goals?*
- *What are the two most important things on my "to do" list? Do them first.*

Worry and anxiety

These sometimes seem like emotional demon twins, with anxious feelings following worrisome thoughts. *Worry* means "to feel uneasy or anxious; torment oneself with or suffer from disturbing thoughts; fret."[7] In the short term, worrying may provide a temporary measure of relief. If it continues, however, it makes things worse for you because it becomes an endless loop, playing your fears and misconceptions over and over in your head. Here's the problem: worry creates the *illusion* that you're working on your problem, when in fact, *worrying accomplishes nothing.*

Worry takes over your mind, tenses your body, drains your energy, and usually ruins your attitude. It makes you feel anxious, distressed, or uneasy because of your fears of what might happen.

TIPS:
- *Set a "worry time," like 3:00 p.m. Sit down then with pencil and paper. Concentrate. Write specifically what's worrying you so you can see it.*
- *Cross off items you have no control over, no power to change. Let these go.*
- *Cross off the trivial items (use Big Deal theory).*
- *DO something about the remaining items. Worry immobilizes you, but activity energizes you.*

Other problems

You chose this one, so in your perception, what is the problem? Write it down. In what ways does it inhibit your opportunity for a *Second Blooming?* List five options for minimizing its impact on you, then choose the two best ones and implement them.

Remember...

As you progress through this book, you'll be reinforced in your efforts and continue to grow strong. The "weed-be-gone" steps you selected in this chapter will also enhance your spirituality, as you'll see next.

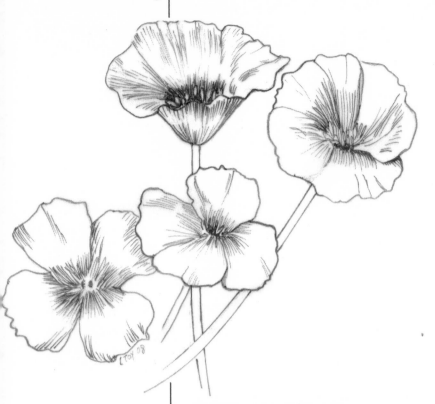

California Poppy

The California poppy is cherished by California Indians, both as a source of food and for oil extracted from the plant. It grows wild throughout the state. Indians also used its pollen as a cosmetic. It's sometimes called "dormidera" (late sleeper) because of its tendency to open its petals later in the morning than most other wildflowers. It's a small plant, with one flower per stem. Yet near Los Angeles, in Antelope Valley Poppy Reserve, a high desert area, the flower covers practically every square inch of the 1745-acre site in spring.

— *State of California Web site*

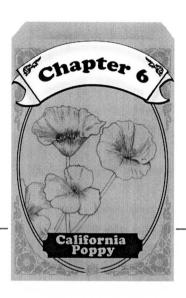

Chapter 6

Organics:
Trust Your
Authentic Self

by Betsy

California Poppy

"This is what I want from now on: a slower pace, a more centered existence, and the feelings of perfect happiness to be found in the moments I come home to myself." ~ Linda Weltner

An organic garden is free from artificial influences and chemicals. In the same way, look at how to rediscover, honor, and trust your natural self. You do not have to reinvent yourself; instead, recognize that you already have everything you need within you for an abundant life. Rather than adding more activities in an effort to embellish yourself, pare down, rediscover, and reclaim vital parts of yourself that have been covered up for years. As you do so, listen carefully to your inner voice because it is your soul talking to you. You've been like a flower bud, held tightly on the tree of life by responsibilities—children, jobs, elderly parents—waiting patiently for your season to bloom. This is it!

Blooming begins with clarification of your authentic self. You can start this process by investigating the role that spirituality plays in your life, and cultivating the self-trust to live authentically.

The role of spirituality

In his book *There's a Spiritual Solution to Every Problem*, Dr. Wayne Dyer quotes the Sufi poet Rumi: "In spiritual consciousness view yourself as a flower in a garden and everyone else in the garden connected to you in some way."[1] This is especially meaningful for you in your second half of life because your spirit is the essence of who you are. Dyer also quotes the ancient Eastern holy book Bhagavad Gita: "You are born into a world of nature; your second birth is into a world of spirit: Spirit represents that which you cannot validate with your senses."[2]

Spirituality plays a role in developing self-trust, but it is not synonymous with religion. Dyer explains that the key to understanding spirituality is the idea of your inner world and your outer world, two unique aspects of being human. He proposes that you think of the physical as a light bulb and the spirit as electricity.[3] The philosophy of my coach training is that you are not a human being having a spiritual experience; rather, you are a spiritual being having a human experience. Spirituality is private and meaningful to each individual and is vital to developing self-trust.

Self-trust

In chapter 4, you explored choices and changes. The next step in preparing for the coming years is to strengthen your self-trust, which is an important element of your life and critical for an abundant *Second Blooming*. In Erik Erikson's eight stages of development, he defines the first stage for infants as *trust vs. mistrust*.[4] When you were helpless and dependent on your parents, you learned if the world could be trusted or not. If you were fed, changed, and nurtured, you developed an attitude of trust. Or, you might have become fearful and learned not to trust if your needs were not met. Self-trust continues to develop throughout life, and you especially want to strengthen and draw on this attribute in your *Second Blooming*.

What is the payoff for self-trust?

We queried the women about this and Beth stated without hesitation, "Confidence. You can own your decisions; you don't have to blame anyone. It's freeing. Independence is beautiful. There are no drawbacks."

Mary added, "If you make a decision that doesn't fly, just learn from it and go on. Not many bad decisions are life-threatening."

"I learned not to be so hard on myself," said Beth. "I made each decision based on what I knew at the time, though I've learned more since then. Aren't you attracted to honest people, those who are just trying to be themselves? Get beyond the idea that you are just a mind and a body. You're so much more than that. You've got a higher self. You know how some people just *are*? They're good. You trust them; they're transparent. Seasoned, reasoned, skilled. Self- acceptance…it seems so simple in them."

In order to develop trust in yourself, you first have to know and understand who you are. You receive messages from many sources, and as you mature, you are continuously developing your sense of self. Other people influence the creation of your self-image, too, with the first messages about who you are coming from your parents and siblings. The person you are today is the compilation of many *conscious* and *subconscious* influences through your life. The person you choose to be in your *Second Blooming*, though, will be the result of *conscious* decisions you'll make about yourself.

After decades as a military officer's wife, for instance, Maripaul found that she had to create a role for herself when her husband retired. "My role used to be defined for me," she said. "I didn't have to come up with one because it was there." She's in charge now, and it's a new experience.

Influences on self-image

Your parents were the first people who influenced your self-image through your genes and in the environment they provided, giving you both direct and subtle messages about who you were. Even today, you hear phrases like "she's all girl" or "she is such a tomboy." Messages like these factor into the person you become.

One of the overt messages from my parents that still rings in my mind was, "You're the big sister and have to take care of your little sister." Such messages are not always direct, but indirect messages are often even more powerful. When my sister was in high school in the 1970s, the principal sent her and two of her friends home because their skirts were too short. They all went to my parents' house to change clothes and my mother was furious. She dressed them all in ballet-length formals and escorted them back the principal's office, where she informed him that he was not to tell "my girls" how to dress. My sister and her friends spent the rest of the day in class in their formals. Whether you find this story humorous or appalling, this message was not a "lesson" that she taught us; however, it was a clear message about self-image. Today, both my sister and I clearly exhibit a defiant streak in our personalities influenced by our mother's personality and actions.

Beth told us, "I learned to trust myself at fifteen because of family conflict. I knew to follow my heart but had difficulty as an adult due to pent-up anger. I pushed religion out of my life. When my beloved father-in-law died, I began my spiritual pursuit through meditation, reading, and other means, and eventually became a Buddhist. Within Buddhism, I commit, contemplate, and embrace trusting myself." Beth's experiences influenced her to investigate new practices and beliefs. Certainly, this can occur within your religion, too. Are you open to exploration and expanding your spirituality?

Influential messages also come from siblings. My younger sister, Molly, did not talk much until she entered first grade, and I am sure it was because I talked for her until she went to school. When someone would ask her name, I would answer for her. She was as shy as I was gregarious.

According to Dr. Robert Needleman, birth order influences the development of personality, too, so evaluating your place in the family can be one helpful means of discovering your authentic self. Children in families take on roles. Often the oldest child is the "good" child, the leader, and the responsible one. First-born children often strive to be perfect. Middle children have a less well-defined role, often making a place for themselves outside the family.[5] I have observed middle children playing the role of intermediary between other siblings and parents. Dr. Needleman identifies youngest children as easygoing, spontaneous, and attention-seeking.[6] Only children frequently have characteristics of the youngest and oldest child, both capable and attention-seeking.

Other relatives influence your development, too. You may have a favorite aunt, uncle, or cousin after whom you modeled your behavior. My grandmother loved fishing and I learned to enjoy it as well. In my childhood, I often rode to church with my uncle who was always early.

Following his example, I am always early to any event.

As you matured, there were other influences on self-development, too. I'm sure that you remember how all the girls wanted to be part of the "in crowd" in high school. In college, friends and teachers influenced social as well as academic development. In the first half of life, especially during the "responsible" years, children and spouses often help define our roles, behavior, and activities.

Self-esteem

Self-esteem affects everything you do and is essential to thriving as you grow older. It is your psychological lifeblood, the fertilizer for your soul. Other ways to describe it include the terms *self-worth*, *self-image*, or *self-confidence*. It's an attitude of self-acceptance—of appreciating, enjoying, and valuing who you are. And it does not come from acquiring more material stuff; you cannot buy your way into a solid sense of self-esteem.

Women with high self-esteem feel and look good because they reflect an inner security. They care about other people, too, making them feel good about themselves, as well. Like a positive attitude, self-esteem doesn't protect you against life's troubles, but it does keep you more buoyant and better able to deal with life's ups and downs.

Sources of self-esteem

If it's so important, where does self-esteem come from? It derives primarily from four sources, including *family* and *other people* as discussed above. In addition, *fate*—both good and bad—plays a role. Perhaps you're disabled in some way, whether by birth or accident, but fate also let you live in a country where women have rights and are no longer legal possessions.

The best news is that, at this stage of life, *you* are in control of your self-esteem. You can make your own decisions about how to respond to fate or to others' comments. You can choose to accept (if helpful) or reject (if not helpful) their input.

Like many women, you may be hanging on to a poor self-image decades after you've outgrown it, so reassess and update the picture you have of yourself. One woman, for example, said, "By the end of my marriage, I was at such an incredibly low point, I made an appointment with a psychologist. My sessions with him made me feel good again. I was in my forties then." She continued to purposefully build her self-esteem, to become "whole" in the years before she remarried.

If you are to bloom fully, you must believe in yourself. It's a necessity, not a luxury. You will need that inner strength to pursue a meaningful life in spite of negative comments or cultural influences you'll encounter.

Clean out your spiritual garden shed

Tools are important to growing a bountiful garden, and unless you've moved lately, you probably have lots of them in your garage or garden shed. If a hand shovel broke, you bought a new one but never threw out the old one. When plants became root bound, you repotted them, stacking the old pots in the shed "just in case." An inventory of my own garden stuff includes: one strong rake with metal prongs for smoothing the garden bed; a leaf rake missing a third of its fingers; three hand shovels, only one of which I use; four pruners, one good; two buckets for mixing; three bags of expired plant fertilizer; one useless wheelbarrow; and a half-dozen pairs of gloves, only one without holes. Obviously, it's time for me to clean out the shed, putting useful things in order and getting rid of the rest. I'm more productive when there's less clutter.

Metaphorically, think of your life as a "garden shed" issued to you at birth. With every passing year, it has become fuller and fuller, and the seams are about to pop. Messages from childhood are in there, such as let the boys win at games; girls become nurses, not doctors; you're very talented musically; girls don't need to go to college; you're very pretty; we know what's best for you. *Shoulds* and *oughts* take up a lot of room, too, as in, you should be able to have or do it all; defer to your husband's wishes; stay at home when your children are little; help at your child's school; get a degree. It has all gone in, but have you ever taken everything out to see if it's still useful or valid? It is time now to unclutter your life's shed, tossing out what no longer serves you well, keeping only what is valued and uplifting to you. In the process, you'll begin to reveal your inner self, your spirit, and make room for your *Second Blooming*.

"I like your idea of 'shedding,' that we've been covered up with responsibilities that kept us from looking inside ourselves," Beth told us. "I am there, inside."

To develop your inner life, you must nourish it. Just as you require physical exercise to keep your body fit and healthy, so do you need spiritual exercise to prepare yourself to do the things you believe in, to live a meaningful life. The form that it takes is up to you and may involve prayer, reflection, reading spiritual books, or meditating, for example. A deeper understanding of yourself and your place in the world expands your spirituality.

Authentic self-trust is essential to cultivating a life that matters after fifty. Yours will continue to increase as you discover your personality, talents, and strengths in the next chapter.

> Love you
> Love others
> Love life
> It is yours
> ~ Shelby Miller

ACTIVITIES

Critique your behavior, not yourself. Say, for example, "I made a mistake, but I choose to learn from it, not beat myself up."

The purpose of meditation is to quiet your mind. One preliminary practice taught for thousands of years is to count your breaths from one to twenty-one. Then start over again.

Practice meditation or quiet reflection each day for thirty-two days. Go to your favorite quiet, comfortable, and secure place. It may be your sofa, your patio, or perhaps a place in a park or at the beach. Close your eyes and take five slow, deep breaths to clear your mind; then focus on your spirit, the inner you. Begin with ten minutes and expand the time to twenty minutes by the end of the thirty-two days. To remind you of its importance, schedule this time in your calendar just as if it was an appointment with your hairdresser or doctor.

Rose

The rose is undoubtedly the best-loved flower and most widely planted shrub in temperate parts of the world. Centuries of hybridizing have brought us the widest possible range of form and color. Growing roses is not difficult, provided you choose types and selections suited to your climate, buy healthy plants, locate and plant them properly, and attend to their basic needs—water, nutrients, necessary pest and disease control, and pruning. Despite the delicate appearance of their blooms, roses are often quite resilient plants.

— *The Southern Living Garden Book, 359*

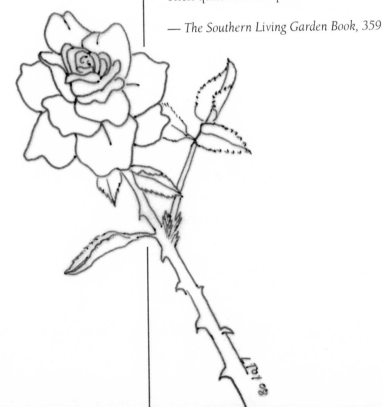

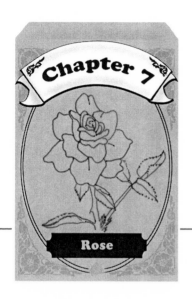

Chapter 7

Rose

Perennials: Appreciate Who You Are

by Kathleen

"Whether we are poets or parents or teachers or artists or gardeners, we must start where we are and use what we have. In the process of creation and relationship, what seems mundane and trivial may show itself to be a holy, precious, part of a pattern." ~ Luci Shaw

You were gifted at birth with a singular selection of personality, talents, and strengths, which like perennials in your garden, provide the foundation for your life. Over the years, perennials may become unappreciated, overgrown, or stunted for lack of care. This chapter will highlight the wonderful characteristics you possess but probably take for granted because they've always been a part of you.

Think of your most prized flower vase. Why is it special to you? Is it the memories it invokes? The traditions? Its shape or artistry? It may even have a chip or two, but still you treasure the vase, which glows from use, burnished by your hands gently holding it while arranging bouquets.

You are like your vase, perfect even in your perceived imperfections. Your personality is your vase, set at birth but revealed over time by experiences, nurturing, and maturity. By the end of this chapter, you'll have a vase full of "roses" representing your many talents and strengths. Together, they make you uniquely qualified to live the life you have been given. You will know yourself in a way that perhaps you never have. Expect to feel affirmed, energized, maybe even surprised, and begin to see why and how you'll thrive in your *Second Blooming*.

In section A, we'll consider personality because it is a biological given; it's your temperament, a set of inclinations, hardwired in you.[1] In section B, we'll look at talents, which are also biologically based, including such abilities as perfect pitch or good hand-eye coordination. In addition to those familiar kinds of abilities, "Talents are your recurring patterns of thought, feeling, or behavior," which determine how you see and interpret the world.[2]

We'll address strengths in section C. According to psychologist Martin E. P. Seligman, Ph. D., strengths are more buildable than talents, as well as more voluntary, measurable, and acquirable.[3]

Dividing the chapter into sections A, B, and C also allows you to pause, reflect, and savor your discoveries.

Considerations regarding personality, talents, and strengths

Betsy and I once more gathered the women. When we asked them to name their top three strengths, it took a couple of quiet minutes before Beth responded with, "Happy, smart, open." Shelby said, "Faith, friendship, loyalty," and Shirley said, "I'm a good friend; I have a good sense of humor." We prodded Mary who finally admitted, "I want someone else to tell me what they are!"

Do you feel like Mary, unsure what strengths are and which you possess? Many of us have spent decades nurturing our children's and spouse's talents, strengths, and dreams, while sometimes neglecting our own. As my artist friend, Anne, said, "I know my husband's strengths better than mine." When I asked her to identify her own, she said, "I don't know. I'm becoming a lot more conscious of my weaknesses right now," yet I see a woman who's creative, caring and compassionate, faithful, and generous. She reflects the challenge we all face to affirm ourselves as we grow older.

Why don't we know and honor our personality, talents, and strengths? Perhaps:

- we weren't encouraged to do so;
- we were busy helping other people;
- we have a false sense of modesty;
- we were brought up to hide our capabilities.

Regarding the last possibility, Anne recalled, "It wasn't a good idea to let the boys know you were smart. It was best to keep quiet."

Beth agreed, saying, "We grew up with, 'You must defer to the male so he can feel better than you.'"

Betsy mused, "How perverse that we had to dummy ourselves down."

No more. It's your turn to bloom, so get ready for a thorough inventory of the perennials in your life's garden.

SECTION A: Personality

"She has a great personality." What does that mean? Does it tell you anything substantial about the woman? Surely we can be more specific in our descriptions. I was quiet and studious. My four siblings were quite different: Bob, a rebel and troublemaker; Carol, outgoing and popular; Hugh, mischievous and entrepreneurial; Stuart, clever and caring. Same parents, different personalities.

What were you like as a child? Do you have siblings? How would you describe them or other family members?

One way of looking at your personality is to assess the kind of person you think you are. Below is a list of adjectives. Look it over, choosing at least fifteen words you think best describe yourself. If you prefer, you can print a copy of this list from our Web site:

www.secondbloomingforwomen.com.

Personality characteristics

Pick at least fifteen words on the following page that you think describe your personality. Work quickly, giving yourself about five minutes. You can add words at the bottom if you want.

practical	idealistic	stable	reliable
introspective	leader	temperamental	loner
playful	imaginative	courageous	curious
nurturing	indecisive	helpful	sensitive
friendly	consistent	responsible	calm
excitable	trusting	jealous	trustworthy
ambitious	mischievous	creative	obstinate
energetic	enthusiastic	emotional	independent
fearful	rigid	intelligent	follower
procrastinator	organized	perceptive	worrier
conscientious	sensitive	clever	quiet
talkative	kind	restrained	anxious
serious	aggressive	open-minded	optimistic
impatient	articulate	poised	confident
dependable	fun-loving	patient	compassionate
conservative	outgoing	sincere	loyal
spontaneous	deliberate	decisive	opinionated
action-oriented	goal-oriented	analytical	expressive
listener	unreliable	pessimistic	genuine

_____   _____   _____   _____

You can also ask someone else who knows you well to pick fifteen words that, in his or her opinion, characterize you. Compare the list with yours. Are they close, or is there a gap between how you see yourself and how the other person sees you? Just notice it for now; there's no need for analysis or concern.

Can you change your personality?

Seligman says that hundreds of psychological studies "converge on a single point: roughly 50 percent of almost every personality trait turns out to be attributable to genetic inheritance."[4] In other words, you're half hardwired.

Despite this knowledge, Marcus Buckingham found that fully 66 percent of us believe the myth, "As you grow, your personality changes." He says the truth is, "As you grow, you become more of who you already are," with your underlying personality remaining constant over time.[5]

Personality, then, can become more evident, given your nurturing and environment, but cannot be rewired. "As you grow, your goal should not be to transform yourself, to somehow conjure new forces from within you," says Buckingham. "Instead your goal should be to free up and focus the forces already there."[6]

In the nature versus nurture argument, research affirms the dominant role nature plays. Change your personality? No. Continue to uncover it? Yes.

How can you learn more about your personality?

Another way of looking at personality is with the Keirsey Temperament Sorter (KTS-II), one of the most widely used temperament sorters in the world. Keirsey identified four basic temperaments, including: Guardian, Artisan, Rational, and Idealist. Each of these has four subtypes, for a total of sixteen personality or "Character Types."[7]

The KTS-II self-assessment tool is included in the book *Please Understand Me II*. It is also available online at no cost; you can complete the seventy-question survey in about ten minutes, and immediately receive the results with a helpful description of your personality. To identify your personality type:

- Google www. keirsey.com;
- find Keirsey Temperament Sorter II, the free online personality test;
- as requested, fill in your name and e-mail address, remembering your password;
- click "Take the KTS-II" Personality Assessment;
- choose "The Classic Temperament Report" which is unlocked and free.

Which temperament are you? Was the description a good match for how you see yourself? Which words or phrases particularly caught your attention? Was there any overlap between this and the fifteen-plus adjectives you chose?

It identified my temperament as Guardian. As a group, Guardians are, for example, helpful and dutiful, with a strong work ethic; cautious and deliberate. Among other things, Guardians also make "loyal mates, responsible parents, and stabilizing leaders."[8] They are concerned citizens and law-abiding individuals.

If you also wish to identify your subgroup and receive more in-depth information, you have the option of ordering from four additional reports for a fee.

I chose to order two extra reports, learning that Guardians split into four subgroups: Inspector, Protector, Provider, and Supervisor, and I'm a Protector. The description is very specific, starting with "Wanting to be of service to others, Protectors can find great satisfaction in assisting the downtrodden."[9] Currently, I'm a member of the local Poverty Solutions Team whose vision is to cut poverty in half by 2020 in our county. Do you think my volunteer activity is a good match for my personality type?

If you do order your subtype, use the description to look at your commitments and activities, and begin to evaluate whether what you're doing is a good match for your personality. This assessment process will continue throughout the book.

How does knowing your personality type help you?

It was affirming for me to see my "type" described so thoroughly and positively. Yes, I'm quiet, but I'm a good listener. No, I'm not spontaneous, but I am dependable. Guardian-Protectors are workhorses and a real asset to their communities—good, solid, essential citizens. In other words, I have value and can appreciate myself as I am. What did you find affirming in your personality type? Which words or phrases resonated with you?

Knowing your type can also help you find a career or field of interest that fits you, something at which you are likely to be successful and also find satisfying. It provides clues to your learning style, as well, since individuals learn best in different ways, such as visually, orally, written word, or hands-on.

Impact on relationships

Personality type affects how we interact with other people, too. Let's look at Betsy's and my relationship, for example. Betsy was identified as an Idealist. Among other things, "Idealists, as a temperament, are passionately concerned with personal growth and development. Idealists strive to discover who they are and how they can become their best possible self—always this quest for self-knowledge and self-improvement drives their imagination. And they want to help others make the journey."[10]

What did this mean for our working relationship? Writing this book was a perfect fit for Betsy's goal of helping others continue to grow. Her enthusiasm was inspiring, keeping me motivated. Coaching as her new post-fifty career is also a good choice.

While I worked steadily, chapter by chapter, Betsy could picture the finished book and describe it in such detail that women said, "I need that book. Where can I buy it?" But she relied on me, the Guardian, to keep us on track. While she was the optimistic cheerleader, I was the practical partner, saying, "Betsy, we have to write the book before we can sell it."

My husband, on the other hand, is a Rational, one who tends to be "pragmatic, skeptical, self-contained, and focused on problem-solving and systems analysis."[11] Rationals are even-tempered and make reasonable mates. The description of Rationals also says they "show love by not holding onto their partner too tightly. They give their partner lots of freedom to pursue their own ideas and dreams."[12] Flack was completely supportive of my writing this book, even asking at times, "Why aren't you writing today?"

You, too, may find clues to important relationships in your personality analysis. If you can encourage someone significant in your life to take the test, you may stimulate some interesting conversations. Topics for discussion might include: What kinds of interactions are typical for our types? What special needs does each of us have? How can we meet these needs as we plan the future and make changes? What kinds of support or resistance might we encounter? What can we both do to help this relationship flourish as I create my *Second Blooming*?

Personality summary

You are special, born with a temperament that allows you to see and work in the world in your unique way. Temperament is hardwired with a set of inclinations. That's the nature part. Then, within each Character Type or subgroup, an individual "unless blocked or deflected by an unfavorable environment, will develop the habits of character appropriate to his or her temperament."[13] That's the nurturing part. There's no need to try to change or transform yourself; instead, claim and reveal your own personality in the coming years. Be yourself.

SECTION B: Talents

Now it's time to see what "roses" your lovely vase holds, and the first ones we'll look at are your talents. Like personality, talents have a biological base, and they can be both physical and mental.

There are several other words for talents, including ability or capability, forte, knack, bent, endowment, natural or innate capacity, aptness, faculty, aptitude, proficiency, gift, and proclivity. Choose whichever words you like, but they all describe biologically based gifts which endure over time.

As Seligman says, "Talents are more innate. For the most part, you either have a talent or you don't; if you are not born with perfect pitch or the lungs of a long-distance runner, there are, sadly, severe limits on how much of them you can acquire."[14] I recall a wonderful neighbor whose degree was in music. In addition to playing the piano expertly, she often sang perfectly executed solos in church, but she was missing the biological gift in her vocal chords to add special richness. She had maximized her talent; no matter how great her desire or how many voice lessons she took, she would never "sing like a bird."

At the other extreme, when I was in my thirties, my husband and I were at the home of some friends. There were about thirty people present, including some from out of town. Danny, our host, asked a young woman to sing while someone else played the piano. Reluctantly, she did, and I was astonished. "She sounds just like Helen Reddy," I whispered to Flack. Years later, I asked Danny if the singer had ever done anything with that powerful voice. "No," he answered, "she was too shy." It was a talent that languished.

When you're young, development of your talents depends on a variety of factors, such as nurturing parents and teachers, a supportive environment, your personality and level of motivation, self-confidence, and enthusiasm. Which of these might our young "Helen Reddy" have been missing? Which were present or missing for you as you grew up?

Now as an adult, it's your choice whether or not to use your aptitudes, to do what's necessary to bring them to full bloom. Jot down at least ten talents you possess. Areas to consider include music, art, dance, sports, math, literature, science, machinery, construction, etc. One approach is to start with, "I've always been good at _____," or, "Other people tell me I'm good at _____."

Other kinds of talents

Another way of looking at talents is offered by Marcus Buckingham and Donald O. Clifton, Ph.D., in their book *Now, Discover Your Strengths*. In addition to physical talents such as running fast, they identify talents as "your naturally recurring patterns of thought, feeling, or behavior."[15] They say it isn't just our physical talents, but also our mental ones that are pre-wired, i.e., the ways we see and interpret the world around us. Buckingham and Clifton's study by the Gallup International Research & Education Center interviewed more than two million people over twenty-five years in their systematic examination of excellence. Looking for patterns, they identified thirty-four themes of human talent.[16]

Their book is an in-depth exploration of how our brains work regarding talents, why it's important to be aware of our talents, and how to use them to develop and build our strengths. If you choose to purchase the book, it has a printed code, which allows you to go online, take their profile (approximately thirty-five minutes), then receive your results with all thirty-four personal themes ranked from strongest to weakest.

An unexpected change and an explanation

When I first wrote this chapter, people could also go online, take the Clifton StrengthsFinder inventory, and learn their top five themes for free. That has changed, however, and now the inventory is only available by buying a book which provides an access code for it. This was not a change I anticipated, so, as we talked about in chapter 4, I've had to adapt. It was never my intent to cause readers any extra expense or effort by purchasing *Second Blooming*, but given the current situation, here are some options for you to consider:

• Buy *Now, Discover Your Strengths* by Marcus Buckingham and Donald O. Clifton, Ph.D., published in 2001 by Free Press. It will have a code for the 1.0 version of StrengthsFinder. (Caution: book must be new as the code in used books will not work.) The book is available in bookstores.

• Buy *StrengthsFinder 2.0: A New and Upgraded Edition of the Online Test from Gallup's Now, Discover Your Strengths* by Tom Rath, published in 2007 by Gallup Press. The book can be purchased in bookstores, or from the Gallup store at: https://store.gallup.com/ They do offer quantity discounts for ten or more copies. (Again, book must be new for the code to work.)

• Buy a used book or check out a copy from the library. Although the code won't work, you can read the descriptions of the thirty-four themes, deciding which ten sound most like you. Narrow the list to your top five. This won't be as accurate as taking the online inventory, but will still be helpful and is fascinating reading. Actually, I did this before taking the test with an accuracy rate of approximately fifty percent.

• Disregard the inventory, continuing with the rest of the book. When we refer to talents, use the ones you identified earlier in this chapter.

Rather than interrupting the flow of your work if you do want to purchase or find a book, you can temporarily skip the rest of this section on talents, moving on to Section C and even chapter 8. The results of the StrengthsFinder inventory will be used again in chapter 9.

Examine your results

If or when you do have the StrengthsFinder results, read your profile. Do you agree with it? Were there any surprises? Which themes were ranked higher or lower than you expected? Have you been using the top talents in your life, whether at work or elsewhere? If not, why do you think they've been rarely used or dormant?

How do these themes play out in life?

Let's begin to explore this by looking at my own themes:

Strategic – #1. This is my #1 signature theme; remarkably, it's also Betsy's #1. We see patterns where others see complexity, and we like to work on a conceptual level. "What are the basic principles?" we ask ourselves. This theme also allowed Betsy and me to plan and visualize the entire book in the form of a proposal.

Responsibility – #2. If I commit to doing something, you can count on me to complete it. "This conscientiousness, this near obsession for doing things right, and your impeccable ethics, combine to create your reputation: utterly dependable."[17] Working on my own, I might never have finished writing this book, but with Betsy counting on me, there was no way I would let her down.

Learner – *#3*. I took a two-year writing course. For *Second Blooming*, I've read dozens of books and hundreds of articles. In my volunteer work, I'm learning a lot about poverty—its causes, effects, and possible solutions.

Connectedness – *#4*. This one reflects my soul, beliefs, and values, and directs all that I do. My philosophy of life is that we are all part of the larger humanity and must care for and respect each other. *Second Blooming* is one way to connect with women, a means for us to share our lives.

Intellection – *#5*. The description of this one made me laugh out loud: "Wherever it leads you, this mental hum is one of the constants of your life."[18] My brain is always working. Intellection also means I like my time alone to contemplate and create. Even with Betsy, we talk and plan, then work on our own.

For comparison, let's look at Betsy's themes:

Strategic – *#1*. It's probably what brought us together, this dominant talent.

Maximizer – *#2*. The description says, "You don't want to spend your life bemoaning what you lack. Rather, you want to capitalize on the gifts with which you were blessed."[19] Betsy seeks excellence in the community, in her business, and in helping individuals. Encouraging growth is exciting to her.

Futuristic – *#3*. Betsy could see *Second Blooming* in the bookstores two years before it was published. She envisioned radio and television interviews, magazine articles, and the seminars we'd conduct. She keeps hope alive.

Relator – *#4*. Betsy and I weren't close friends when she asked me about writing a book; more than anything, we were business acquaintances. She took the initial steps to deepen our relationship and build on our common talents, strengths, skills, and dreams.

Positivity – *#5*. Betsy's fun to be with, and she's full of enthusiasm and possibilities. She sees what's positive in people and situations, and her excitement keeps everyone motivated.

As you can see, Betsy and I complement each other. Her *futuristic* and *positivity* themes keep us upbeat, while my *responsibility* theme keeps us on task.

You may want to encourage someone close to you to take the Clifton StrengthsFinder Themes profile, too, and then have a discussion about your personal or working relationship based on your outcomes. What do you have in common? Where do you differ? What strengths does each of you bring to the relationship? What do you value in each other?

Implications of themes for choice of jobs and activities

What impact do these talents have on your everyday life? For starters, if you're still in the workplace, be aware that Buckingham and Clifton's research found, surprisingly, "Eight out of ten employees feel they are miscast. Eight out of ten employees never have the chance to reveal the best of themselves."[20] Are your talents being used in your position? Do you feel productive, positive, and fulfilled by what you are doing? Are your top talents and job requirements a good match? If not, is there any leeway for you to restructure your job to emphasize your themes? Might you brainstorm with your boss or co-workers and swap some responsibilities for a better fit, benefiting both you and the organization? If you can't restructure your job to use your talents, perhaps you need to consider a career or job change. You shortchange both yourself and the organization if you don't feel like you're a good match.

The following is one way to see if you're putting your talents to good use. First, list your primary activities. Next to each one, decide which of your top five talents are used. The example below lists a few of my activities (some real, some not). For each activity, write down which of my talents, if any, it uses. The first two are done for you.

Activity	Talent(s) it uses
Cooking and serving food at a soup kitchen on Thursdays	connectedness
Member of small local writers' group	learner, intellection
Working to eliminate poverty in county	_____
Sales position with local newspaper	_____
Social Club: plan social activities for the year	_____
Do training for Big Brothers Big Sisters staff	_____
Plan fund-raiser for Symphony Orchestra	_____

Were there any activities that used none of my talents? If so, what recommendation would you make to me? What are the possible consequences to me for continuing to be involved in activities that do not use my talents? Did any use several talents? What do you think that means?

Now make a similar list with your own activities. Again, you can print a form to use at www.secondbloomingforwomen.com.

Activity	Talent(s) it uses
_____	_____
_____	_____
_____	_____
_____	_____
_____	_____
_____	_____
_____	_____

Are you involved in any activities that don't use your top themes or talents? If so, is there a compelling reason (such as honoring your commitment) for you to stay involved, at least for now? What was your motivation in taking on the activity? Is it still valid?

Another approach to assessing how or whether you use your talents is to show your top themes to some people close to you, asking such questions as:

- Do you see me using these talents?
- In what ways?
- In your opinion, am I doing anything that doesn't match my theme talents?
- How might I put my talents to better use?

Keep everything you're learning about yourself together. It's not time to make decisions or take action because we're going to look at strengths next. And as Buckingham and Clifton note, "These themes of talent may not yet be strengths. Each theme is a recurring pattern of thought, feeling, or behavior—the promise of a strength."[21] In other words, talents are raw materials that develop into strengths with practice, knowledge, skills, and experience.

Treasure your talents, remembering that not everybody can do what you may find obvious or easy. You are uniquely gifted.

SECTION C: Strengths

Your strengths are less biologically dependent than personality and talents, and therefore more malleable. In fact, they are changing even as you grow your way through this book.

But first, a little theoretical background. For most of my professional life, psychology focused on identifying and classifying people's problems, like depression or paranoia, and trying to fix them. Counselors looked at what was wrong with people and tried to help them change, to become more "normal." Such was the career of Martin E. P. Seligman, Ph.D., too, until he was elected president of the American Psychological Association in 1998. He had a vision, a radical idea at the time, of taking psychology in a new direction, "to look at what actively made people feel fulfilled, engaged, and meaningfully happy. Mental health, [Seligman] reasoned, should be more than the absence of mental illness. It should be something akin to a vibrant and muscular fitness of the human mind and spirit."[22] The academic field of Positive Psychology developed quickly under Seligman's leadership, and you and I are the beneficiaries of his and others' research.

In *Authentic Happiness*, Seligman describes three levels of happiness, all of which have validity and a necessary place in our lives. Here's my brief summary of his view: [23]

Happiness level	**meaningful life**
Focus	meaning
Uses or employs	signature strengths and virtues in service of something larger than self
Examples	work to eliminate poverty

Happiness level	**good life**
Focus	engagement
Uses or employs	signature strengths in main realms of your life
Examples	care for elderly parents; work

Happiness level	**pleasant life**
Focus	pleasure
Uses or employs	senses; emotions
Examples	take a bubble bath; enjoy a delicious dinner; feel gleeful

Obviously, "happiness" has a quite a different definition than many of us are familiar with. Instead of the transitory, feel-good experience of a bubble bath, authentic happiness is deeper, longer-lasting, and more meaningful. You already know what gives you sensory pleasure, such as a massage or a child's kiss on your cheek, but I believe you bought this book because you also want more of the good life and the meaningful life. For those, you need to develop and use your strengths. But what are your strengths? How can you identify them?

Identifying your strengths

If you purchase *Authentic Happiness,* it includes detailed descriptions of the twenty-four strengths as well as self-assessments and explanations of results. Another option is to go online to take the Values-in-Action (VIA) Survey of Character Strengths at no cost. (When I first took the survey, it was called VIA Signature Strengths.) You are asked to provide some basic information about yourself, and upon completion, you will immediately receive results ranking and describing your specific strengths. Registration and your chosen password allow you to revisit the site as desired, taking the survey again later to see if your strengths have changed, reflecting your personal growth.

There are several other interesting surveys at the same site, such as the Meaning in Life Questionnaire, but first take the VIA Survey of Character Strengths which measures twenty-four character strengths so you can begin to use the results. There are several ways to access the questionnaires and surveys, but you can follow these steps:

- Google www.authentichappiness.sas.upenn.edu;
- you will see several categories of interesting questionnaires, including the featured questionnaire, emotion, engagement, meaning, and life satisfaction questionnaires;
- under "engagement," look for VIA Survey of Character Strengths which measures twenty-four character strengths; click on the survey;
- log in with your name (or e-mail) and a password you choose;
- take the VIA Survey of Character Strengths (240 questions which take approximately thirty minutes).

After you've done that, look at your strengths. The top five are considered your "signature strengths." How do you feel about them? Were there any surprises in the overall rankings? Any disappointments? In your opinion, what do your top five strengths say about you right now?

Before we continue with your strengths, let's look at Betsy's top five, which were:

- humor, playfulness;
- zest, enthusiasm, energy;
- bravery, valor;
- creativity, ingenuity;
- hope, optimism, future.

Knowing only this much about Betsy, could you in good conscience recommend that she become an accountant, secretary, bank teller, or lawyer? Would those careers take advantage of her signature strengths? As a theme, it appears that she needs to work with people in positions requiring "out-of-the-box" thinking and a positive vision for the future. She needs a constantly changing, challenging, and invigorating environment.

Now, reflecting on your own signature strengths, what themes or trends do you see? What kind of environment are you most likely to thrive in? Do you need people or projects? Activity or quiet? For what kinds of things are you *not* suited? Are you a good match for what you're involved in right now? Have you gained any insights?

Accepting your strengths

Do you accept your strengths and their ranking, or do you wish for another outcome? You'll recall Mary saying earlier that she wanted someone else to identify her strengths, so I invited her to take the VIA survey. She did, and her signature character strengths were:

1. judgment, critical thinking, and open-mindedness;
2. capacity to love and be loved;
3. forgiveness and mercy;
4. gratitude;
5. honesty, authenticity, and genuineness.

Mary's reaction was mixed. "I wish my strong suits (#s 2, 3, and 4) weren't so geared to that whole gentle side of life." But she has lupus, so she added, "I don't like that lack of zest and energy, but that's the way it has to be. I just hate that's it's gone."

"What," I asked, "the physical energy or the mental energy?"

"Both," she replied. "Number 21 (zest, enthusiasm, energy) wouldn't have been that low before my illness. Now my mind is tired."

"What were you pleased with in the assessment?" I asked.

Mary thought for a moment. "I especially liked #1, judgment, critical thinking, and open-mindedness. I value that highly. Numbers 2, 3, and 4 are *so* related. I guess I wanted some "pop" in there, some more active stuff. I certainly value #5."

I felt compelled to tell Mary how much *I* valued her top strengths.

"Don't you remember when Flack had his cancer surgery? You were at the hospital by 7:00 a.m. and stayed with me for hours until they wheeled him out of the operating room. That was an incredible gift to me."

"Well, I guess." She didn't sound convinced, so I continued, "Did the VIA survey results encourage you to make any changes in how you value yourself?"

"It encouraged me to make some changes with #20 (self-control, self-regulation). I'm already working on #21 with various exercise programs."

I pursued the issue. "I sense you're still focused on your weaknesses instead of your strengths."

"Yes, I think I am. I'm not sure how to go out and light the world on fire, but I'm feeling more energetic than 2, 3, and 4."

Circumstances affect how you use your strengths

Mary retains a mental picture of her strengths before developing lupus and caring for her mother, a picture at odds with the strengths she shows now. The challenge to Mary and to you? To value all of your character strengths, but especially your top five signature strengths. Understand that they may change over time depending on your health and other circumstances. If, like Mary, you're not too keen on your top strengths, ask some family or friends how they see you using them in a positive way. As Shirley said, "Somebody else sometimes scratches the surface to let those strengths out."

Focus on strengths or fix weaknesses?

"You will grow the most in your areas of greatest weakness," many of us have been told over the years. In *Go Put Your Strengths to Work,* though, Buckingham says that's a myth.[24] But how easy it is to picture parents looking at their child's report card, scanning the grades, skipping over the As and Bs without comment, then asking, "What's this C in math? You need to bring up that grade." As adults, we take on that role for ourselves, saying, "That's an area I need to work on."

Buckingham stresses, "You will grow the most in your areas of greatest strength."[25] Seligman concurs, "I do not believe that you should devote overly much effort to correcting your weaknesses. Rather, I believe that the highest success in living and the deepest emotional satisfaction comes from building and using your signature strengths."[26]

Fill your vase

In working through this chapter, you've identified your personality type, top talents, and signature strengths. Now it's time to arrange them in a bouquet so you can appreciate your unique beauty. Draw a picture of your own treasured vase, or print one from:

www.secondbloomingforwomen.com

with five roses to the left for talents and five to the right for strengths. Write your personality type on the front of the vase. (Mine is pictured, for example.) See how special you are? Be proud of yourself.

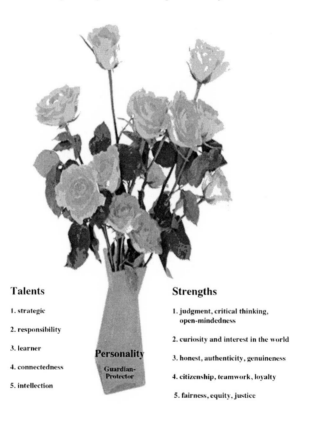

Talents

1. strategic

2. responsibility

3. learner

4. connectedness

5. intellection

Personality

Guardian-
Protector

Strengths

1. judgment, critical thinking, open-mindedness

2. curiosity and interest in the world

3. honest, authenticity, genuineness

4. citizenship, teamwork, loyalty

5. fairness, equity, justice

But isn't that bragging?

Absolutely not. Bragging is when you feel and promote yourself as being superior to other people, whereas an honest self-assessment lets you understand and appreciate your uniqueness. Accepting your many gifts will let you make positive, productive plans for your life.

In the next chapter, you'll fill out your bouquet with "annuals," the skills you've developed over the years.

ADDITIONAL RESOURCES

Please Understand Me II: Temperament, Character, Intelligence by David Keirsey, Ph.D.

Now, Discover Your Strengths by Marcus Buckingham and Donald O. Clifton, Ph.D.

Go Put Your Strengths to Work by Marcus Buckingham.

Authentic Happiness by Martin E. P. Seligman, Ph.D.

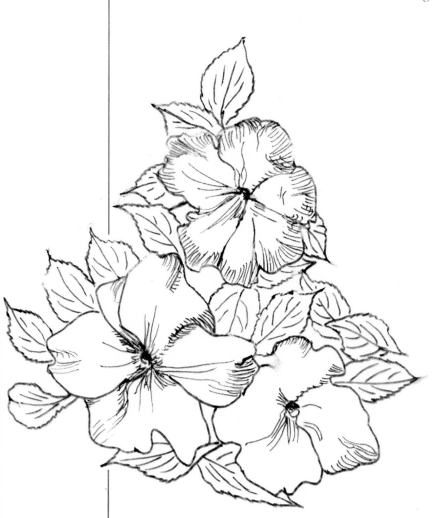

Impatiens

Impatiens does everything well and asks little. It's marvelously adaptable in shaded or semi-shaded landscapes, and blooms prolifically from spring to late fall in beds, borders, pots, or hanging baskets. Strains exist in bewildering variety. All types produce months of bright color. Ripe seed capsules burst open when touched lightly and scatter seeds explosively. Plants often reseed in moist ground.

— *The Southern Living Garden Book, 255*

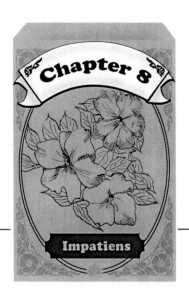

Chapter 8

Impatiens

Annuals: Inventory Your Skills

by Betsy

"Life is so constructed that we move through different phases and stages, each requiring the skills and wisdom of the previous ones." ~ Anne Wilson Schaef

"Summer snapdragon Angelonia angustifolia, is one of the hottest new summer annuals in the market today. Landscape professionals and horti-culturists are raving about its heat and drought tolerance, extended bloom period, and performance in the landscape," announced a gardening e-mail I received. Annuals such as snapdragons and impatiens beautify a garden by bringing color, variety, and a new show every year against the familiar background of perennials. In the same way, you've added skills annually as needed or desired to enhance your talents and strengths. Remember making the move from typewriters to word processors and computers?

Unlike talents and strengths, which are more biologically based, skills can be taught, learned, and often transferred from one situation to another. As Beth said, "Strengths are innate, skills are learned." Learning about and applying your skills will help you know yourself better, live more purposefully, and attain personal satisfaction.

Marcus Buckingham has a formula to show how many of the elements we've discussed so far fit together:[1]

strengths = talents + skills + knowledge

With this chapter, you will understand skills and their benefits, identify your own skills, consider transferring some of them to different activities, discontinue using others, and explore adding new ones.

Understanding skills

Would you believe the average person has five hundred to eight hundred skills?[2] Amazing. How many of yours can you list off the top of your head? I could probably do fifty.

A skill is anything you can do right now. You develop skills in various ways, whether on the job, through hobbies or volunteer work, training or education, and they allow you to thrive in various aspects of your life.

There are three types of skills:[3]

- *Job-specific* skills are necessary for doing particular tasks (e.g., preparing tax returns, filing, telemarketing, editing copy, analyzing budgets, data entry, plastering, operating equipment).
- *Adaptive* skills are also sometimes referred to as self-management or personality skills (e.g., honest, diligent, able to work independently, follow directions well, efficient).
- *Transferable* skills can be used in many different job settings (e.g., handle money, write well, do public speaking, conduct research, solve problems, delegate, train others).

In addition to these three kinds of skills, Connecticut's Department of Labor names a dozen broad categories of jobs:[4]

artistic	scientific	plant and animal
protective	mechanical	industrial
business	sales	service
human service	leading/persuading	physical/performing

Examples are given for each category, which may prove helpful in beginning to identify your skills. At the end of the chapter, in the *Identifying your skills* section, you'll learn how to connect with Connecticut's Web site and several other Web sites.

Benefits of knowing your skills

No, you're not looking to sell yourself as a "product" to get a job, but instead to find your purpose, which may or may not involve employment. What, then, are some of the benefits of assessing your skills?

- Knowing them can provide clues to what you might like to do in the future…or not.
- Talents are the raw materials of your life, but they remain as potential unless you make the effort to acquire the necessary skills. Identifying your current skills may highlight others that you want or need to maximize your talents.
- Skills also allow you to build your signature strengths, bringing your inclinations to fruition.
- It's fun and affirming to see them all together. You are much more skilled than you may think.

Developing skills in your *Second Blooming*

We asked our friends, "Are there any skills you've chosen to develop or grow since you turned fifty?"

Shelby told us about one she's been working on recently—writing. She said, "I never knew I had it in me." When I asked, "What was the trigger that got you started?" she replied, "Not having a full-time job. I wrote letters in the past and people liked them. Then, I had the desire to write. Instead of buying a card, I'd write one. It just flowed out of me. I joined the writers' group and their positive feedback made me keep going." Kathleen and I are honored to have several of Shelby's poems in our book.

Mary told us about transferring her teaching skill from children to adults. "I had always been in front of children. I learned on purpose to be more comfortable in front of adults by teaching Sunday school. It's still a teaching situation, and I'm gaining confidence."

In the course of writing this book, I talked with a friend, Cindy, who is creative with crafts and sewing. We were in her sewing room and I was marveling at her talent, complimenting her work and ordering custom Christmas gifts for my granddaughters. She inquired about the book and shared with me that she was impressed by my creativity with words. That was my first compliment regarding creativity. I consider it a talent, while writing is a skill that I have transferred from graduate school. I used a different style of writing for this book, but I applied my earlier skills.

Seventy-nine year old Betty, a retired school principal, was a model for the Northwest Florida Council on Aging's fund-raising calendar with a grand piano as her prop. The calendar celebrates the beauty of people over sixty. She sat at the piano as if she were playing. Her interest was piqued, so she took lessons and now plays every day and often in the middle of the night when she cannot sleep. Betty's newfound musical skill gives her fulfillment and satisfaction, and brings pleasure to sleepless nights.

I was forty-nine when I became obsessed with the game of golf. I took many lessons, playing at least twice a week. For months, I would schedule a tee time and then dread going due to my inadequate skills. I wanted to play at a level ten immediately, of course, yet I knew I couldn't unless I played often, so I forced myself to get in the cart, tee off, and play. Eventually, the stress lessened and the enjoyment increased as my skills improved with practice. Interestingly, we teach our children to be patient and take learning one step at a time, yet as adults, some of us want to skip the learning and go directly to mastery.

Risks and rewards

According to Dona Lerner, my current golf pro, the key to improving your skill at golf is to risk vulnerability and to be open to failure. You must be willing to evaluate mistakes as you start learning. She also believes many life skills are transferrable to the golf course. Strategic planning is important because the golfer must be able to see an opportunity and plan her shots accordingly. Not surprising, emotional control is a skill that is beneficial to becoming a good golfer. Sometimes, however, women and girls have to be taught how to celebrate their success. Dona's experience has shown her that many women anticipate failure, thus success is unexpected. Yes, even celebrating success can be a learned skill.

My passion for tennis began when I was fifty-seven and my golf obsession paled in comparison to my tennis addiction. I spent untold thousands of dollars on lessons with handsome, young tennis pros who kept me challenged, while at the same time, made me feel competent. During my tennis years, I was the most physically fit ever since I worked out four days a week and played daily. My skills increased rapidly and my body toned quickly. Osteoarthritis in my knee forced me to put away my tennis racquet, but with new golf clubs and a new pro, I'm back on the links.

In each of my sports experiences, I started as a novice, but persistence and practice allowed me to increase my skill level significantly. Golf taught me that most people on the golf course are not at the level of Tiger Woods or Annika Sorenstam who have underlying talent in addition to persistence, practice, and skills. I also agree now with Buckingham and Clifton who found "while skills will help you perform, they will not help you excel."[5]

I accept that I lack the talent to achieve mastery, but my enjoyment and increased self-confidence were worth every sore muscle and every dollar spent.

You may not play tennis or golf, but what new skills have you pursued? What was your learning curve? What kept you motivated? Where else in life were you able to use your new skills?

Transferring and adding skills

You can transfer some of the skills that you have developed throughout life to your *Second Blooming* as Kathleen and I did in writing this book. When I asked what she used in writing it, Kathleen said, "It's the culmination of everything I ever learned and did. I had to pull wide-ranging skills together in one massive effort." As a teacher, she knew how to develop lesson plans, critical to outlining and writing chapters. She incorporated her training and seminar skills into the exercises and examples given in each chapter. She also took a writing course shortly before embarking on this venture to increase her expertise. Kathleen was emphatic: "There's no way I could have tackled this subject until now, in maturity. I didn't have the knowledge or skills when I was younger. Or the guts."

My professional life coaching skills have been useful, too, and many of the questions we posed to our friends came from my coach training. I have developed skills in PowerPoint presentations, blogs, and rudimentary Web sites, and I'll also use the skills I learned while teaching an online course to create online workshops and teleclasses for our readers.

What skills do you want to build upon and transfer to your future? Were you the organized mom who always got the neighborhood kids to events on time? Did friends look to you for decorating ideas or home repairs? Have you always served as the social hostess? Were you the unofficial confidante and counselor for friends? What did other people call on you to do? In other words, what skills did they recognize in you?

Retiring Skills

One great thing about this age is being able to say, "Been there, done that." When I asked Beth, for instance, "Is there a difference in the skills you use now compared to when you were thirty-five?" she said, "Way different. I see myself snipping off the extraneous stuff. For example, I want to retain the knowledge base of nursing, but not the 'doing,' like giving intravenous medications."

Kathleen developed the skill of "cold calling" on organizations to sell employee assistance program contracts in one of her jobs. Although she never liked it, she became proficient at closing the sale because she was committed to the value of what she was doing. She gladly released cold calling from her duties when she was able to hire another person to manage the business aspects of the job. Then, with this new person on board, Kathleen could build her delegation skills.

One of the most difficult roles in my career was as the negotiator at the collective bargaining table. I was a good one, although I hated every second of it. I retain the skill, though it is seldom required in my second half of life, and I will not seek ways to use it.

Looking ahead, Deb said, "It's always been important to me, climbing the career ladder, but now I want to let go of the responsibilities of being boss. I know how to supervise, but I don't want to do that anymore. I want to just worry about me and my part."

You, too, can give yourself permission to let go of skills that you don't want to use anymore, focusing instead on the ones you enjoy or find beneficial for your own purposes. When you release old skills that are not helpful or appealing in your second half of life, you open up opportunities to gain new ones or use old ones in new ventures.

Identifying your skills

There are several ways of identifying your skills. It doesn't matter which method you use, only that you make an effort at gathering your skills in one place so you can appreciate how competent you are, assess which ones you might like to transfer to future activities, and pick the ones you'd like to cut out of your life. You can try any or all of these methods, which I found by using the key words "identifying skills" on Google.

- The Connecticut Department of Labor's Web site is useful for getting started. Visit www.ctdol.state.ct.us/progsupt/jobsrvce/skills.htm for examples of job-specific, transferrable, and adaptive skills. For each of the dozen broad categories we mentioned at the beginning of the chapter, it provides examples of associated skills.

- Utah's Occupational Information Network Web site www.online.onetcenter.org/skills/ has lists for various kinds of skills, including: basic, complex problem-solving, resource management, social, systems, and technical. It's one page with a quick checklist. When you're finished, you can click on 'Go' to see how your skills match up with specific occupations. Some matches will seem bizarre to you (e.g., my top match was 'sales engineer'…no way) but overall you may get an expanded idea of areas of interest to which your current skills may be applied.

- Georgia's Department of Labor Web site www.dol.state.ga.us/js/replace/chapter04.htm helps you group your skills into categories by using a Skills Triangle. You can also view and print lists of Transferable, Self-management, and Job Content Skills for easy use.

- Minnesota's Department of Employment and Economic Development Web site www.deed.state.mn.us/cjs/cjsbook/skills1.htm provides a written process if you prefer a more analytical approach. It explains steps 1–3 in more depth:
    1. list the titles of jobs (paid or volunteer) you have had.

2. list 4–5 major tasks or functions required to perform each job.
3. list all the skills needed to accomplish the tasks.

- If you have no interest in using the computer or just want one more way to assess your skills, here's my approach. Using the following list of skills:
    1. highlight all those you have right now;
    2. place the letter **L** beside any you might want to learn in your second half of life;
    3. place the letter **T** beside those you want to transfer to your future;
    4. place an **X** beside those you want to retire.

SKILLS

Sewing	Painting	Writing
Acting	Running	Softball
Swimming	Tennis	Golf
Knitting	Drawing	Cooking
Gardening	Weaving	Photography
Organizing	Delegating	Singing
Storytelling	Playing a musical instrument	Telling jokes
Crocheting or Knitting	Biking	Motorcycling
Horseback riding	Teaching	Coaching
Conflict Resolution	Entertaining	Engaging
Strategic Planning	Public Speaking	Editing
Listening	Communicating	Assessing
Analyzing	Strategizing	Coordinating
Follow through	Counseling	Manager
Learning	Boating	Sailing
Foreign Language	Decorating	Politics
Attending to details	Planning	Repairing
Fashion	Jewelry making	Collaborating
Flower arranging	Tutoring	Training
Selling	Negotiating	Having Fun
Business building	Making connections with people	

Imagine that you are completing the bouquet you began in chapter 7. You are surrounded by buckets of beautiful flowers—your skills. Pick those that will fill your vase with the most color and brilliance. By creating this bountiful bouquet of talents, strengths, and skills, you have prepared yourself for clarifying your passions and dreams in chapter 9.

ACTIVITY

Look over all of your skills from all of the lists, circling a dozen or so that intrigue you, energize you, or you simply enjoy using. These are more clues to what you'll want to do in your Second Blooming.

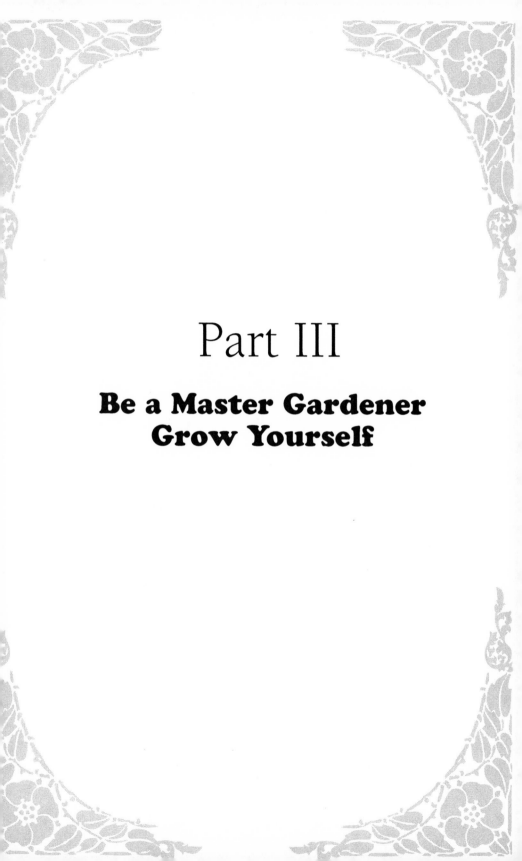

Part III

Be a Master Gardener
Grow Yourself

Rocky Mountain Columbine

The state flower of Colorado, the Rocky Mountain columbine, is an early-summer flowering plant. It's one of the easiest perennials to grow with a delightful, interesting flower shape. It is a versatile, cultivated wild flower, delightful to find along a wilderness path.
The name is from a Latin word "columba," which means dove, as the flower looks like the bird of peace. It grows from Nova Scotia to the Northwest Territories and continues south into areas of Florida and Texas. Rocky Mountain columbine is noted for the bell-shaped flowers and fragrance. Its shape makes it well suited for attracting long-tongued nectar feeders, especially hawk moths and hummingbirds. It also has a rich history in the herbal market.

— *State of Colorado Web site*

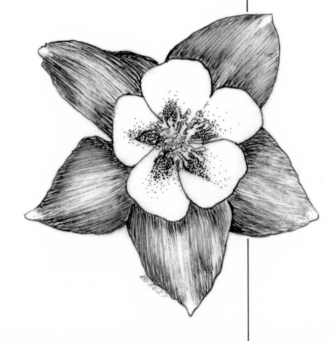

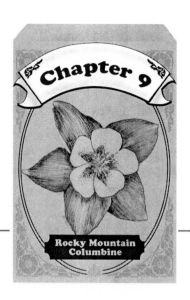

Rocky Mountain
Columbine

Decide What to Plant: Clarify Your Passions and Dreams

by Kathleen

"As the season of believing seems to wind down, let me gently remind you that many dreams still wait in the wings. Many authentic sparks must be fanned before passion performs her perfect work in you. Throw another log on the fire." ~ Sarah Ban Breathnach

Why do you exist? Can you complete this sentence? My purpose in life is to _____. If you can, wonderful; if not, you will by the end of this book. The next three chapters will continue to guide you in that delightful process of self-discovery.

Some women are born knowing their life purpose. My sister, Carol, always knew she'd be a nurse. Other women, like me, evolve over long periods of time, constantly experimenting, reassessing, and reevaluating. I've often thought how much easier it has been for Carol with her single-minded passion, but then I'd have missed the exploration and adventures that culminated in writing this book. For a few women, their life purpose comes as a revelation. In 1999, for example, one woman took a vacation by herself, heading to Ecuador where she volunteered in a daycare center for indigent and handicapped children. Her goal was to conquer the fear of going alone; instead, she found her purpose. "The entire course of my life changed after those two weeks. For the first time in my life, I felt useful—and realized that each of us is born with an inherent desire to serve."[1] Ever since, she has encouraged and helped others to find their service passion, too.

What is purpose?

Purpose is your sense of direction in life, living out your dreams, measuring up to your potential, and awareness of it can come in different ways. Some women's faith may provide them with guidance or mission. For instance, a friend called to ask me about becoming involved in eliminating poverty in our county. "I just feel like God is calling me to this issue," she said.

Put simply, your purpose is what you were born to do. It means living an authentic life, using all of your unique talents, strengths, and skills for something meaningful, whether in your family, at work or church, in your community, or in the larger world. It doesn't have to be huge or world changing, just important to you. It's also being true to your nature, and not copying someone else. I can admire other women such as Eleanor Roosevelt and author Maya Angelou, but if I try to emulate them, I'll fail. The same is true for you. The only and best person you can be is you.

But my life is full already!

You may well be thinking, "My life is very full, so why should I bother with this purpose stuff?" Consider carefully: Is your life full of meaning, or full of activities? If you didn't have a deep need for meaning, acknowledged or not, I don't think you'd be reading this book. Trust your intuition because as we said in chapter 6, it's your soul calling out to you: *I hunger, I yearn for meaning.*

You probably know women who are drifting through life aimlessly, busying themselves with various activities so they can't hear their heart's whispers. Sadly, they are the women who, at the end of their lives, will be lamenting, "If only…" or, "I wish I had…" or, "If I could live my life over, I would…"

There are also more immediate and practical consequences to living without purpose:

• Drudgery is one. Work is harder without heart.

• You empower other people and circumstances to shape your life by default; in other words, you'll be a follower of someone else's dreams and decisions.

- You won't know when to say yes or no to requests for your time and energy.
- You'll react to things rather than being proactive, which may result in frittering away your life on trivia.

If that's not how you wish to live your remaining years, there's hope. Keep reading.

Benefits from knowing your purpose

By contrast, there are many benefits from knowing your purpose:

- It simplifies your life because it helps you make decisions on what to do or not do. For example, a friend called recently, saying, "Kathleen, I know how much you love music, so I'm inviting you to become a member of the Symphony Guild. We have a number of interesting activities and fund-raisers." Because I was clear on my purpose, I was able to decline politely but firmly. You won't need to make up lame excuses, either, for saying no.
- It helps you be a better time and life manager by concentrating your thoughts and energy on what's important. You can't do everything, so you'll select what has value to you.
- You will also be able to distinguish between activity and productivity. Do you sometimes get to the end of the day thinking, "I was busy all day, but what did I really accomplish?" Purpose will help you choose and prioritize meaningful activities.
- A clear purpose gives you motivation and energy, a reason to get up every morning and anticipate the day. You'll want to continue to learn, experience, and grow.
- It enables you to deflect criticism and get around obstacles. In the midst of writing this chapter, for instance, we received yet another rejection letter from an agent. The last time that happened, I quit writing for two weeks. This time, I just tossed the letter in the "Agent" folder and said out loud, "Too bad for you. It's going to be a great book." And I kept on writing.
- Purpose lets you lead an authentic life. You'll feel at ease with yourself and the world, at peace, whole. "It's a feeling of being who you were meant to be, of being fully human and alive and unselfconscious while you do your work."[2]

- It also reduces stress. The greater the gap between who you truly are and what you're doing, the greater your stress. As you narrow that gap, stress diminishes, which is good for your physical and emotional health.

So my life will be easier

Not necessarily. In fact you may work harder than ever, but the rewards of satisfaction, joy, and authentic happiness will be well worth it. When the Northwest Regional Director for the Make-a-Wish Foundation was asked why she did it, she said, "It is so rewarding. It's the best and hardest thing I have ever done."[3]

By now you may be wondering, "If a life purpose is so important, what's keeping me from finding what mine is?" To answer that question, start by becoming aware of significant external and internal factors. As you read next about various external and internal issues, ask yourself with each one, "Is this factor playing a role in my life?"

External influences

- *Materialism.* We live in a society that seems to value things over meaning. All day, every day, we are bombarded with images and advertisements promising Love! Beauty! Health! No pain! If we'll just buy designer clothes, an upscale car, more cosmetics, the latest medications, new furniture and appliances, granite countertops. Buy, buy, buy, they tempt us. Nan Adams, one of my church's ministers, gave thoughtful sermons over three weeks on this issue. She said, "That's the myth—that happiness, fulfillment, peace in our souls comes from acquiring *things*, and especially those things that seem to be in short supply."[4]

- *Our upbringing.* No matter how educated, liberated, traveled, or experienced we are, we retain vestiges of our upbringing, and for many of us, those were times when men were bosses and women were their secretaries. In learning to write, if we were talking about an individual, "he" was used; there was nary a female pronoun to be found. With some exceptions, our expansive youthful dreams were channeled into becoming secretaries, nurses, or teachers, or otherwise limited by society. My sister recently met a woman at a University of Michigan alumnae luncheon who graduated in 1964, the same year I did. Carol wrote me: "The woman stated that she was excellent in math and while in high school, she discussed economics with her father who suggested that she apply to U of M's business school, which she did. After graduating, she became a Certified Public Accountant (CPA) and applied for positions with accounting firms. Most of the rejection letters said, 'We do not hire women.' Only two firms offered her a job. One stated that if she accepted a position with their firm, she would be assigned to tax returns as their clients were not ready to have a woman manage their investments." It's time for us to banish those old, artificial boundaries on our aspirations.

• *Timing.* My husband often says, "Timing is everything." Perhaps it's not time quite yet for your *Second Blooming*. You may still need to work, for example, to ensure your financial future. One friend never married and is totally self-dependent, so she continues working at a job that doesn't match her purpose because she needs the good pay and benefits. You may have other responsibilities, too, such as a disabled adult child or sibling, or grandchildren who need you. Maybe you're a caregiver, like Mary is. Even if it's not time now, you can begin preparing so you're ready to bloom later. Deb, fifty-two, estimates she has several years yet to work full time, but says, "Now's the time to start and make progress."

• *Relationships.* Whether intentional or not, there may be people who don't want you to dream, to change, to replant your life's garden, because any shift you make requires a shift in them, too. When one woman wanted to get a job, her husband said pointedly, "You can do anything you want, as long as nothing changes at home." Another was attending some self-awareness sessions at a church other than her regular one. "I feel happy and whole when I'm here. So why are the people closest to me, my family and friends, against my attending?" she asked the people in her small group

Internal issues

External factors certainly play a role, but even more important is what goes on inside your head. And that's good news, because you have a lot more control over it. Some of the major issues include:

• *Procrastination*. Do you find yourself thinking, "Well, there's always tomorrow. I'll do it then"? That outlook may work up to age fifty; after that, we become aware that there's more life behind us than ahead of us, and we feel a growing urgency to use our time well. After nearly two years of trying to land an agent, for instance, Betsy and I decided to take control of the publishing process because, at best, it would have been two more years until publication. "At this age, I'm not willing to wait that long," I told her. "I want to hold this book." One of the women's conversations touched on this theme, too:

> Mary: Do you ever have an idea of what you want to do, but it doesn't fit right now? Do you put it off, or do you act?
>
> Beth: I usually act. If I'm interested, I do it till it fizzles out.
>
> Betsy: There's a Zen saying: Leap, and the net will appear. Don't put it off. We're not going on thirty anymore.

(You can refer back to "procrastination" in chapter 5 for more information.)

• *Guilt*. As adults, we lived for decades in the "responsible" growing zone, nurturing our family at home and perhaps building a career at work. However, it can be difficult to go from selfless to self-oriented without experiencing some guilt. Many of us are not accustomed to saying, "I want to…" or "I choose to…" At first, it can sound and feel selfish, so practice saying it out loud every day. You'll get used to it. Remember, it's your turn to unearth your passions and dreams. (See guilt and regret in chapter 5.)

• *Self-confidence*. Is your little inner voice protesting, "But I'm not good enough, smart enough, capable enough, worthy enough to have dreams"? Tell it to *hush!* Life is not a contest in which you compare yourself to other women and come up feeling inadequate. Your personal challenge is to be the best possible woman you can, using your unique gifts to live up to your potential. Confidence is not required to start, just willingness. Confidence will grow with your accomplishments. If you wait until you feel confident, you'll never start.

• *Attitude*. This can pull you down—or elevate you—faster and further than anything. If you accept the notion that you're less and less valuable as a human being with every birthday, you're doomed. Vow now to ignore any people, ads, articles, books, or media that imply so. You're never too old to grow into your amazing gifts of life. If the world won't lift you up, lift yourself. (Revisit chapter 3, if appropriate.)

• *Fear.* This can be a major stumbling block. If you've always been a logical person, accustomed to using your head, you may fear following your heart and instincts as you try to discover your purpose. Or maybe you treasure your safety, comfort, and security, wondering why you should change things at this age. (Reread chapter 4 on Change as needed.) Finding your purpose also usually involves risk, which many women find disconcerting. "But what if I fail?" you ask. You won't. You can't. You can only fail if you don't try. When you're gone, do you want people to say, "She lived a safe life" or, "She lived fully?" It's your choice. A wonderful line in an obituary read, "She died doing the life she loved."

• *Unknown passions and dreams.* After one of our first presentations, a woman confided to us in a note, "I have no idea when I started losing enthusiasm, feeling overwhelmed, not really able to remember what my dreams might have been." In her forties, her life was directed by the needs of her family and the demands of her job. Sound familiar? As in a winter garden, your passions and dreams lie dormant, and by your fifties, you may no longer be sure what's underground. Like bulbs, though, your dreams are awaiting their season to burst forth in colorful abundance. It's time to let those bulbs poke through, time for you to bloom. Dreams don't have expiration dates.

Uncovering your passions and dreams

For most of us, our purpose isn't evident, and discerning it takes time. You can begin to clarify it through self-discovery and experimentation, starting with a look at your passions and dreams. Over the years, some of them have been buried, a few thrown on the compost pile, while others are waiting to be planted and take root.

Passions are strong feelings or "compelling emotion; strong fondness, enthusiasm, or desire for something."[5] The word "compelling" especially indicates that true passion cannot be ignored or buried easily; it insists on being acknowledged—sometimes in spite of our efforts to squelch it. Intense passion demands action. As author Charlotte Bronte said, "I am just going to write because I cannot help it."[6]

Dreams are closely related to passions, but have a more ephemeral nature, floating free-form through your mind. There are the dreams when you're sleeping, which can sometimes provide clues to your passions and purpose. Random House Webster's College Dictionary describes these as "a succession of images, thoughts, or emotions passing through the mind during sleep." Of more interest is "an involuntary vision occurring to a person when awake." This may be an "Aha!" moment for you, when what was working in your subconscious suddenly pops into consciousness and you can clearly see your future. What a gift! Accept it with gratitude.

Other dictionary definitions of dreams include "to conceive; an aspiration; goal; aim; a wild or vain fancy; most desirable; ideal," but my favorite is "to imagine as possible."[7] That's the goal of this chapter: to inspire you to picture your passions and dreams as possibilities.

Why are dreams important?

And what role do they play? The women responded to these questions:

Mary: There's something about a dream embodying hope.

Beth: Dreams feed the imagination.

Shirley: They're just good for you. I think you need to dream. It gives your mind and body a rest. You sit; your mind wanders…sometimes goals come up.

Mary: They can put you in touch with a deeper layer.

Shelby: I think for me a dream is forward-looking, not behind. It gives me a reason to continue, to hope, despite changes in health. I need a dream so I can contribute by using my mind.

For Deb, "Dreams also help us deal with disappointments and problems in life. Disappointments happen to everybody. Having that dream for the future can help bring you back from the edge, the black hole. It helps you hope."

How do I uncover my passions and dreams?

First, start by becoming conscious of what you're doing, thinking, and feeling as you live each day. Have your journal with you constantly for at least the next week so you're ready to capture fleeting insights. In addition, schedule some quiet time every day. Choose a quiet spot, with no music or other distractions. You may not be able to do this at home since that's your workplace and the temptation to succumb to activities— answer the phone, do the dishes, fold the laundry—is strong. Allow the silence to talk to you and share its secrets. It may take a few days before you stop being twitchy and begin to hear your inner musings more deeply.

Trust your body's signals

As part of the "I can't afford to get sick because I have to take care of everybody else" syndrome, we're often not in tune with—or simply ignore—our bodies, missing vital clues to our passions and dreams. Start to pay close attention to what you're doing or thinking when you experience certain:

physical clues, such as:
- your heart beats faster;
- you feel physically more alert;
- you're energized by an activity instead of drained;
- you possess greater strength or endurance than usual;

emotions and feelings, including:
- pleasure or joy;
- satisfaction or fulfillment;
- confidence;
- pride;

mental or thought processes when:
- acquiring new knowledge or skills comes easily;
- you actively seek other ways to use this new information;
- you lose track of time when engaged in the activity.

Stimulate your self-discovery

To help prompt your self-discovery, respond to the following questions. You don't have to reply to all of them, just those to which you have an immediate or visceral reaction. You may have several responses to some questions, and none to others. (Betsy, for example, had no reaction to questions 8–10 and thinks that may be because she never had children.) Leave your head out of this, trusting your heart and gut by jotting down what comes to you first. You'll have a chance later to ponder what it means. Use small slips of paper; sticky notes would be even better so you can move them. Put only one response per slip, along with the number of the question. You can also print these questions from our Web site www.secondbloomingforwomen.com.

To help identify passions, respond to:

1. I feel excited and energized when _____.

2. I feel angry and upset when _____.

3. I'm fascinated by _____.

4. I'm drawn to magazines and books about _____.

To help identify dreams:

First, dig up your youthful dreams…

5. When I was a little girl, I wished I could _____.

6. I especially loved _____.

7. As a teenager, I pictured myself _____.

Then recall your "responsible" years…

8. I used to enjoy _____, but I had to give it up because _____.

9. Despite my responsibilities, I was still able to _____.

10. I put _____ on the back burner.

Now, as a woman over fifty…

11. If money were no object, I'd _____.

12. People would think I'm crazy, but I'd like to

_____.

13. If I just had the time, I'd _____.

14. If I knew I were to die next week, I would most regret

_____.

15. I want to be remembered for _____.

Deciding what to "plant" in your life

It's time for some fun. First, label four blank sheets of paper as shown below.

A. passions	B. dreams to let go	C. dreams to keep	D. passionate dreams to explore further

Next, look at your stack of responses to questions 1–4 (identifying passions). Stick the slips on sheet A (passions), spreading them out so you can see all of them.

For each dream (questions 5–15), ask yourself the following questions, and depending on your answer, put each slip on sheet B (dreams to let go) or C (dreams to keep).

- "Is this my dream or someone else's?" For example, who wanted you to become a dancer, you or your mother? If it's not your dream, let it go.

- "Does this dream still fit?" When I was ten, I was crazy about horses and everything to do with them—books, games, statues, riding—but that was a phase I'm finished with. If a dream no longer fits you, let it go.

- "Does this dream need to be updated?" Perhaps you wanted to become a doctor, but that wasn't feasible when you went to college. Are you willing to go to school now in the medical field? Or volunteer at a clinic? Work at a hospice? Write medical articles? What options do you have for activating this dream? If the options appeal to you, keep the dream; otherwise, let it go.

Now you have sheet C with "dreams to keep." Look it over thoughtfully to see if there's a match or connection with any of your passions on sheet A. Choose those dreams that evoke your passion, energy, and sense of purpose, and move their slips to sheet D (passionate dreams to explore further).

What did you learn about yourself in this process? Were there any surprises? Is there anything you need or want to add to any of the sheets? This may take place over days or weeks. Just looking at sheet D may be enough for you to see what direction you want your life to take. Terrific! If not, or you just want to think about your passions and dreams in another way, the method that follows can help.

Further exploration

If you tend to be more analytical or want to understand your gut feelings better, here's a process for pulling together everything you've learned about yourself this far so you can look at it objectively. You will need:

- your notebook or journal containing your personality type, top talents, signature strengths, and the descriptions of each from chapter 7;
- your skills list(s) from chapter 8;
- sheets A (passions) and D (dreams to explore further) from chapter 9;
- a block of time to work, perhaps an hour.

As you read these steps, you can refer to the two examples which follow before using them for your own dreams.

1. Choose a dream from sheet D (passionate dreams to explore further). Write it at the top of the "Assessing Passions and Dreams" chart (a blank one will be provided later for your use).
2. In the first column, write down which passion(s) from sheet A the dream invokes.
3. Under "Suits my personality," write your personality type (Guardian, Artisan, Rational, or Idealist), and subtype, if you ordered it. This came from section A in chapter 7. From the personality type description(s), choose several characteristics you possess that will help you achieve this dream.
4. Also from chapter 7, section B, look at your top five talents from the Clifton StrengthsFinder Themes profile (or your best estimate of them). Of these, choose which ones will be needed to fulfill this particular dream.
5. In chapter 7, section C, you took the *Authentic Happiness* Values-in-Action (VIA) Character Strengths Survey to identify your top five signature strengths. In the fourth column, write down which of the strengths will be used.
6. Lastly, look at your skills, deciding which you already possess that will be used in achieving this dream. In your opinion, which additional skills might you need to acquire?
7. Ignore the last "values" column for now, as it will be addressed in chapter 10.
8. Choose a second dream from sheet D and repeat these steps.

Assessing Passions and Dreams: Example #1

My dream is **to write and publish a book for women**

Invokes my passion for...	Suits my personality...	Uses my top talents...	Uses my signature strengths...	Skills I have or can learn...	Matches my values...
Helping people enrich their lives	Yes. As a "'Guardian-Protector," I am: helpful, responsible, grounded, and happy working alone. I want to be of service to others. I seek belonging to a group or community.	Strategic (can see patterns in complexity) Responsibility (conscientious, ethical, dependable) Learner (energized by learning) Connectedness (as women, we're all connected, want to build bridges among us, caring and accepting) Intellection (reflective and introspective)	Judgment, critical thinking, open-mindedness Curiosity and interest in the world Honesty, authenticity, and genuineness Citizenship, teamwork, and loyalty (doesn't use fairness, equity, and justice very much)	Already, I: can write clearly; can organize complex thoughts; took an advanced writing course; know how to accept feedback; am in a writing group; am able to use computer; wrote proposal and query letters. Need to learn more about publishing process: 1. marketing 2. publicity 3. using blogs and Web sites	

Assessing Passions and Dreams: Example #2

My dream is to **create stained glass windows**

Invokes my passion for...	Suits my personality...	Uses my top talents...	Uses my signature strengths...	Skills I have or can learn...	Matches my values...
Creativity, art	Somewhat: as a Guardian-Protector, I am: diligent, willing to work long hours, happy working alone.	Responsibility (conscientious; near obsessiveness for doing things right) Learner (love taking classes and learning new things) Other: I have a good eye for color; I do well with precision work.	Curiosity and interest in the world	No skills Don't know what skills I need	

In looking at these two dreams, which do you think I'm more likely to realize? If you were advising me, which one would you encourage me to pursue? Why? This isn't a contest with the dream having the longest columns winning; intense passion, for example, can sometimes override a lack of talent or skills. However, the chart does provide significant visual, thoughtful information to consider.

Now it's your turn. Use this same process for at least two of the dreams that you choose from your "passionate dreams to explore further" sheet D so you can evaluate them. There's also a blank chart you can print at www.secondbloomingforwomen.com.

Assessing Passions and Dreams

My dream is to

_____

Invokes my passion for...	Suits my personality...	Uses my top talents...	Uses my signature strengths...	Skills I have or can learn...	Matches my values...

Keep dreaming and experimenting

Perhaps "passions and dreams" seem too big, too intimidating to you; or your list seems skimpy, as if you've been living in a cave; or you just feel something's missing that you don't even know about. If so, think of topics that interest you, or activities that catch your imagination. Sometimes you have to try new things to even be aware of what you might do. Inspiration can come from unexpected, humble beginnings. A local woman, for instance, wanted an area rug for her new home's hardwood floor, so she decided to hook one. The newspaper reported, "As she spent hours upon hours working on her rugs, she found the handwork was actually turning into a pleasurable activity and it stirred her artistic muse. 'I've always enjoyed working with my hands such as hand stitching or gardening. It was peaceful for me. After getting started, I instinctively knew it was right for me. I was hooked.' "[8] She's now nationally known for both her rugs and her teaching skills.

Beth continues to experiment. "Yes, I'm blossoming. My writing is expanding, but because of Lyda (who did the flower sketches in this book), I'm also learning to paint. And I'm learning quilting from Mary's mom. I don't care about the end product, I just like doing."

As for Maripaul, "I tried several things, but they didn't work, so I kept looking. I'd tell myself, 'Try something new.' "

I encourage you, too, to trust your instincts, follow your heart, and see where they take you. The possibilities are endless and exciting. As you find things that intrigue or tempt you, add them to your "passionate dreams to explore further" sheet.

Some seeds lay dormant
Left to patiently wait
Now my life is unfolding
Surprising, exciting
Passionately surprised
By what was there untended
Until now
~ Shelby Miller

Honor all dreams—past, present, and future

You have identified many of your passions and dreams. Whether you choose to act on them or not, honor and respect all of them because they reflect your wholeness. Appreciate what they tell you about yourself, affirming them as essential elements of your ever-evolving life.

By now, you may sense the direction you want to head. Don't make your final choices on which dreams to pursue yet, though, because there's one more issue to consider, one more column to fill in on the passions and dreams chart: values. In the next chapter, Betsy will help you identify your core values and understand what role they play in your decisions.

Crepe Myrtle

Crepe myrtle is among the most satisfactory of plants for the south, with showy summer flowers, attractive bark, and often-brilliant fall color. It tolerates heat, humidity, drought, and most well-drained soils. It may be frozen to the ground in severe winters in the upper south, but will re-sprout. Crepe myrtle blooms on new wood and should be pruned in winter or early spring to increase next summer's flowers.

— *The Southern Living Garden Book, 267*

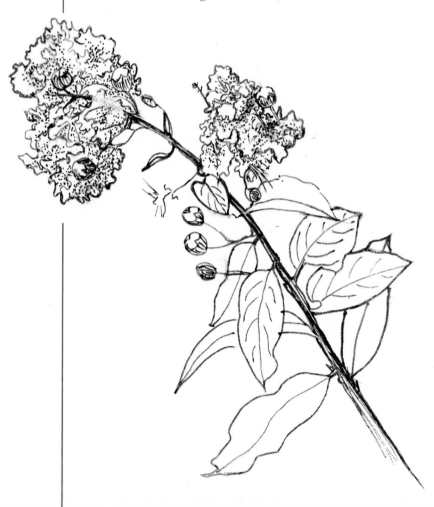

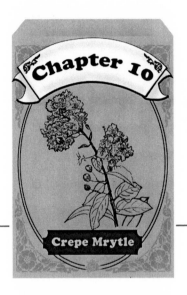

Chapter 10

Crepe Mrytle

Pinch and Prune: Ascertain Your Values and Vision

by Betsy

"Within our dreams and aspirations we find our opportunities."
~ Sue Atchley Ebaugh

Pinching and pruning can make a plant more compact and can also result in a profusion of flowers. Just as pinching and pruning enhance the growth of plants, identifying and clarifying your values enhances growth and achievement of your passions and dreams in your *Second Blooming*.

Why are values important?

Values are your essence. They are the beliefs that guide your every decision, the building blocks of your personal foundation, and the principles by which you live. Your convictions regarding what you believe is important and desirable are determined by your values.

Determining your values

Before you read further, stop and write down the names of three people whom you truly admire and respect. These people can be living or dead, real or fictional. (When I did this exercise with a group of college students, one of them wrote that she admired the engine from *The Little*

Engine That Could.) Next, under each name, list at least three attributes of that person that gain your respect. I've provided you with an example. You will find a complete form for this exercise on our Web site www.secondbloomingforwomen.com.

1. One person I respect is the Honorable Marie Young, County Commissioner, Escambia County, Florida.
2. The attributes I respect in her are:
   • straightforwardness;
   • caring for others, and;
   • sense of humor.

The attributes that you list for these people are, in actuality, your own values. Often it is easier to identify values that are important to us in other people than in ourselves.

You may or may not be conscious of your personal values. Every person has a set of complex values, which may shift somewhat throughout life. Those core values, the essence of you, stay as your foundation throughout life while others may be added or deleted, depending on life experiences.[1] Occasionally values conflict, as when a working mother values both her career and her children.

The following is a list of values, which will assist you in identifying your own values. A more thorough list is located on our Web site www.secondbloomingforwomen.com.

Achievement	Knowledge	Success	Practicality
Adventure	Leadership	Punctuality	Resourcefulness
Competition	Loyalty	Accuracy	Beauty
Creativity	Love	Peace	Self-reliance
Excellence	Freedom	Harmony	Honor
Excitement	Honesty	Fun	Friendship
Family	Competition	Faith	Physical Challenge
Integrity	Pleasure	Decisiveness	Money
Quality	Trust	Justice	Unity
Serenity	Wisdom	Status	Change

Take time now to make your list, beginning with twelve. Of those, identify your top five, and then choose three of the five that are most vital to you. These three are your core values.

As you enter your *Second Blooming*, your emphasis on certain values may shift. Think back to your values when you were in your thirties and forties, the responsible years, and which were emphasized. Family, for example, may have been one of your top values then and you still treasure it today. However, if your children are now grown, you can emphasize it in a different way. Family is still important, but it doesn't consume your every waking moment.

At this time of life, you can choose to reevaluate your values, changing your emphasis on some and even identifying new ones that bring you renewed energy.

How does it feel when your values are not aligned with friends, family, work, community, or other areas of your life? Are you uncomfortable? Do you experience stress or irritation? If so, you may choose to spend less time with old friends or with certain family members. Your interest or passion for groups to which you belong may wane. This is a "wake-up call" to reassess your current values and to realign your second half of life with new goals.

Now you can fill in that last values column in the "Assessing Passions and Dreams" chart in chapter 9.

Know when and how to say yes and no

Your values empower you to invest your time and energy in matters about which you are passionate. You can now say yes to those things in alignment with your core values, and you can say no to those things that are not. Remember, please, no is not a four-letter word. No is a powerful word, but it tends to be used infrequently by women. Since your time is precious, you want to spend it wisely on the things that are important to you and will help you achieve your goals. When someone asks me to take on an activity, I pause and ask myself, "Will this help me reach my goal?" If it will help me, I reply yes; if it will not, my answer is no.

You have the right to say no. Others may take you for granted or even lose respect for you if you always say yes. According to Harriett Braiker, author of *The Disease to Please: Curing the People-Pleasing Syndrome,* if you think you are a bad person when you say no, you may suffer from the "disease to please."[2] Saying yes when you really want to say no leads to resentment in the person making the request and anger within yourself.

She feels let down and disappointed, and you feel guilty.

Ways to say no

There are as many strategies to saying no as there are methods to pinch and prune flowers. Judith Tingley, Ph.D., recommends that no be the first word out of your mouth, followed by a brief reason. She is adamant that you not give several reasons, you do not give excuses, and you do not apologize. A quick "I don't want to go to the movie tonight" is sufficient and communicates that you are serious.[3] Or, you might be willing to negotiate by suggesting that you go to dinner tonight and the movie another night.

Here are some additional ways to say no:

- Saying no after saying yes: "My apologies, but I've overcommitted myself. Unfortunately, I must back out of my commitment." This is effective when you have agreed to a project and then discover it has more responsibilities than originally outlined.
- Diplomatic no: "I'm flattered that you thought of me, but I won't be able to help you."
- Not right now: "I've done it before and hope to do it again, but I can't help at this time".
- Absolute no: "I'm not interested in doing this; I don't have the time or energy."

If you say yes when you really mean no, you appear unreliable, unenthusiastic, or scatter-brained, so pare down your commitments and focus on doing the things about which you are passionate.

Creating your vision statement

Rosabeth Moss Kanter said, "A vision is not just a picture of what could be; it is an appeal to our better selves, a call to become something more."[4]

With dreams, passions, and values clearly identified, you now enter into the creative aspect of personal development, designing your vision, which is the picture of your entire life's garden in bloom. Dreams are the various perennials and annuals that must be planted to make that vision come to life, and passion is the fertilizer that nourishes it.

Your vision is important because it guides your life and has the power of anticipating your next ten, twenty, or thirty years. It is the light that illuminates your path and helps you create a purposeful and powerful life. One of my favorite coaching questions is, "If you could wave a magic wand, what would you create for yourself?" Your vision is magical, created by clearly stating what you want without regard to limitations. This is the time to stretch your brain, your heart, and your spirit. A compelling vision statement:[5]

- is written down; keep it nearby so you can see it frequently;
- is written in the present tense, as if it has already been accomplished;
- covers various topics and activities;
- is descriptive, filled with images, sounds, smells, and people.

Laurie Beth Jones tells us, "Your vision statement is the force that will sustain you when your purpose statement seems too heavy to endure, enforce, or engage. All significant changes and inventions begin with a vision first."[6]

During a conversation with our friends, one of them asked Kathleen and me if we had a vision. We did, and this is how we pictured ourselves five years from then. Note how the statement is written *as if it has already come true.*

> *Second Blooming* has been on the market for five years now and it continues to sell well. We are both speaking at various local and national conferences, as well as conducting workshops and seminars for women across the country. We are frequent guests on radio and television shows. Sales of our accompanying *Second Blooming Workbook* published four years ago are brisk. We continue to gather stories from women who are experiencing their *Second Blooming* for our third book. We receive many requests to write another book for women in their forties so they can be prepared when they turn fifty.

The impact of a vision statement

After an unpleasant business experience, Laurie Beth Jones wrote the following vision statement: "I have clients who delight and cherish me, and who properly value my creative talents and efforts. We are mutually engaged in serving others. My clients come exclusively through referrals, allowing me to be free to devote my energies to creating. They are doing work or offering products that I respect. They pay me well and on time. I have long-term relationships with the people I serve."[7] Her business turned around after she wrote this compelling statement.

Write your personal vision statement now, letting yourself be guided by all that you learned in the previous chapters.

_____

_____

_____

_____

_____

_____

_____

This statement will allow you to focus on what you *do* want and need in your life, and also serve as a guide for your decisions. Knowing where you're going will help move you forward.

The key to manifesting your vision—goals

The key to manifesting your vision is goals. By setting goals, you create concrete plans for achieving your vision. In order for a flower to grow, you must first stick it into the ground so it can take root. Creating your vision is like planting the flower. Setting goals is like letting a plant take root so the bloom will be beautiful and hearty. You achieve your goals through planning, accountability, and results. Goal setting has been part of your life already because you have successfully planned such things as children's school trips, holiday parties, meals, meetings, and projects. You're simply transferring your skill to a new venture.

Think big when you set your goals. In his book *Good to Great*, Jim Collins introduces BHAGs—Big Hairy Audacious Goals.[8] In *Toastmaster Magazine*, Dena Harris likewise encourages readers to set *BAGs*—Big Audacious Goals.[9] Life coaches like me ask clients to set "stretch goals."

You get the picture. If you want to achieve your vision, you must set big goals that are the steps to achieving it. Danica Patrick, the first women to win an Indy Car race, recommends that in order to achieve a big goal, first find out what it takes to get there, then break it into smaller parts. She states, "No challenge is completely overwhelming if it is broken down properly."[10]

A useful goal-setting technique

A popular technique is SMART goal setting. SMART goals are: **S**pecific, **M**easurable, **A**ttainable, **R**ealistic, and **T**imely.[11]

* *Specific* – Just like a good newspaper article, a specific goal answers these questions as necessary:
    Who—is involved?
    What—do I want to accomplish?
    Where—does it happen (location)?
    When—will it be done (my timeline for accomplishment)?
    Which—restraints or issues are there?
    Why—am I doing this (my purpose or benefits from achieving this goal)?
* *Measurable* – How many? How much?
* *Attainable* – Assess your attitude, ability, strengths, and skills needed to attain this goal.
* *Realistic* – Goals can be both big and realistic.
* *Timely* – Set your timeline so you can track your journey to success.

In March 2009, for example, our SMART goal for this book was "*Second Blooming* will be published by July 1, 2009, and we will sell five hundred copies by August 1, 2009."

Stay flexible

Timelines are important to achieving goals; however, we want to emphasize that if a timeline is not met, it is seldom life threatening. Mother's Day in May 2009 was our first goal for publication, but our ignorance of the publishing process and unexpected events in our lives contributed to not meeting that deadline. When we realized that we would not hit our mark for publication, we shifted our schedule and set a new date.

Enlist support

In chapter 7, Kathleen told you that our friends supported us by frequently asking about the publication date for *Second Blooming*. The following information from the American Society for Training and Development (ASTD) shows the importance of having such people involved in your goal setting:[12]

- The likelihood of your completing a goal if you just have an idea is 10%.
- When you consciously decide to implement an idea, there is a 25% chance you'll finish it.
- Merely deciding when you will realize the goal gives you a 40% chance of accomplishing it.
- If you create a plan, you have a 50% chance of getting it done.
- Committing to someone else that you'll achieve the goal increases your likelihood of achieving it by 65%.
- When you have a specific accountability appointment with the person to whom you have made the commitment, there is a 95% chance that you will actually complete the goal.

The lesson? Tell everyone you know what you're doing and they'll help you accomplish it.

What's next?

In this chapter, I've given you several strategies for writing your vision statement and setting SMART goals. Once you do that, your garden will almost be ready to bloom. By pinching and pruning your values, determining your vision, learning when and how to say yes and no, and establishing your goals, you've prepared yourself well for the next chapter—creating your life purpose statement and developing your action plan.

ADDITIONAL RESOURCE

The Path: Creating Your Mission Statement for Work and for Life by Laurie Beth Jones.

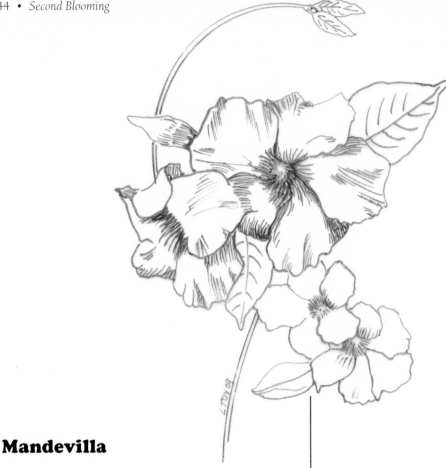

Mandevilla

Mandevilla is a prolific vine that twines around any
structure, and its large blossoms are knockouts. It
also has wonderful foliage. Dark green leaves can
grow eight inches long and three inches wide. Thick,
leathery, and rumpled, they create a coarse-textured
backdrop for the smooth, silky flowers. After it gets
going in spring, mandevilla blooms relentlessly.
Keep it happy by giving it fertile soil and full sun.
Feed it every two to three weeks with water-soluble
20-20-20 plant food. Evenly moist soil is the key.

— *www.southernliving.com*

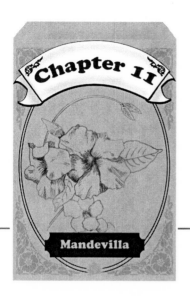

Chapter 11

Mandevilla

Add Water, Fertilizer, and Sunshine: Bring Your Purpose to Life with a Plan

by Betsy

"There are people who put their dreams in a little box and say, 'Yes, I've got dreams, of course, I've got dreams.' Then they put the box away and bring it out once in a while to look at it, and yep, they're still there. These are great dreams, but they never even get out of the box."
~ Erma Bombeck

The next natural step is to tend your garden. You've picked a dream you want to activate and, like a gardener, you can't stop there. It's time to add water, fertilizer, and sunshine to promote peak blooming.

You've reached a tipping point. You're ready to live your purpose, but wishing doesn't make it come true. The next step is to bring your purpose to full bloom with an action plan. It's not so hard. You've probably worked with to-do lists for years and this is merely a step-by-step list, as well. You'll write down specific action steps that will help you reach your goals; prioritize the steps and add dates by which to accomplish them; then, decide how you'll hold yourself accountable and on track. You will overcome roadblocks with a clear focus and purposeful actions.

Life Purpose

Kathleen introduced life purpose in chapter 9 by asking you to complete the sentence: "My purpose in life is to _____." Whether you were able to complete the sentence or not, I encourage you to participate in the exercises in this chapter to affirm your purpose and to develop your action plan. At this point, you've identified your dreams and passions, vision and values, and the roles they play in creating your purpose statement. We do not differentiate between a "life purpose statement" and a "life mission statement" in this book. Whatever you name it, it's the reason you exist. Ideally, you will find yourself saying, "This is what I was meant to do."

Steps to writing your life purpose statement

A good life purpose statement is inspiring, exciting, clear, encouraging, and specific. It covers your personal and professional life, and however you compose the statement, it is just right for you.

My original statement was one long sentence: "My purpose in life is to enjoy the risks of new and rewarding life experiences, to enjoy the challenge of accomplishing new dreams, and to enjoy warm and loving relationships." Whew! It took me weeks to create this with the assistance of my life coach, and I was bemused at the elements of risk-taking, challenges, and joyfulness.

Recently, though, during a mastermind meeting with two fellow coaches, I had an epiphany about my life purpose and my new statement is: "To help people acknowledge their greatness." Short and simple.

Kathleen said her life purpose is: "To motivate and guide adults in recognizing, valuing, and maximizing their potential."

You'll find other examples of life purpose statements later in the chapter. The one you create for yourself now is the beginning step in developing your life purpose, and probably not the final product. Just as you took the time and the energy to identify your dreams, passions, and vision and values, you now want to take time to create and to clarify your purpose statement. One of the following exercises should enable you to do this.

Life purpose exercise #1

This first exercise asks you to select verbs and nouns that are significant to you, and then turn those few words into your purpose statement. Here is a brief list of verbs to get you started. A more exhaustive list is on our Web site www.secondbloomingforwomen.com under "purpose."

First, choose three verbs that are meaningful to you.

accomplish	affirm	alleviate
build	communicate	compute
connect	create	direct
educate	encourage	excite
facilitate	give	implement
inspire	lead	mediate
model	motivate	persuade
produce	pursue	realize
relate	serve	translate
validate	work	write

The verbs that I choose are: _____, _____, and _____.

It's fine if you only have two verbs; if you have more than three, pick the most important ones.

Second, select the person(s), organization, or cause from the list below that will benefit from your life purpose. Again, you will find a more comprehensive list of nouns on our Web site www.second-bloomingforwomen.com.

women	men	youth
infants	creative people	teachers
retirees	new professionals	veterans
disabled people	divorced people	new mothers
elderly	poor	animals
executives	environment	health care providers
boomers	business people	religion
civil rights	government	immigration
music	travel	sports

_____ _____ _____

The group, cause, or organization I want to focus on is: _____. Be specific. If you choose "youth," for example, narrow it down: What age? Are they average? Delinquent? Disabled? Achievers? Creative? Athletic? Shy?

Third, what is it you want to do or have happen with the people, cause, or organization? What's your goal? Again using youth as an example, is your goal with them to increase reading skills, stay out of trouble at school, graduate from high school, help them create an art portfolio, decrease obesity, enhance physical fitness, or start a children's choir? My goal is to_____.

Put it all together in a statement

Insert your words in to this formula: My life purpose is to _____(verb),_____(verb), and _____(verb) _____ (noun/who) to _____ (verb).[1]

Our "youth" example might be: My life purpose is to
- model, inspire, and educate (verbs);
- middle school boys (people, cause, or organization to benefit);
- to meet the president's guidelines for physical fitness (your goal).

When you put it all together, it reads: My life purpose is to model, inspire, and educate middle school boys to meet the president's guidelines for physical fitness.

If I had done my own statement using this process, it might read: My life purpose is to inspire, encourage, and coach women to live a life that matters. Note, too, how closely this statement aligns with my earlier one, which was "to help people acknowledge their greatness." If you try each of these exercises, you will see consistency in the outcomes.

Life purpose exercise #2

The next exercise draws from your history of successes and fulfilling experiences.

1. Write short stories, a few sentences about times in your life when you felt fulfilled. Write and write until there are no more stories. This may take a few hours or several days, but put a deadline of one week to complete it.
2. Read the stories and highlight key words that are alike or repeated.
3. Compose one sentence integrating as many of the highlighted words as possible.
4. Compose your life purpose statement from those words.

Using this process, my own examples of stories or sentences might include:

- I felt fulfilled when I *taught* my class.
- I loved it when I was the keynote *speaker* at the national conference.
- I feel excited when I see people learn their *strengths*.
- I am enthused when my clients reach their *dreams*.

The words that stand out to me are teach, speak, strengths, and dreams, so my purpose statement might have been: "My life purpose is to teach people how to discover their strengths and help them reach their dreams." Notice that this, too, is consistent with my earlier statements.

Now write your life purpose statement:

_____

_____

_____

Experiment as needed

One of these exercises may work perfectly for you, or a hybrid might be your preference. I would not have been able to identify my purpose and write my statement without my life coach; however, Kathleen created hers with no such assistance. You may find *Second Blooming* to be an adequate coach for you, but if not, I encourage you to contact a credentialed life coach to work with you; work with a close friend, colleague or clergy; or use Laurie Beth Jones' *The Path: Creating Your Mission Statement for Work and for Life.* The point is to develop a statement that allows you to live consciously and purposefully.

Examples of life purpose statements

By looking at various women's statements within one field of interest—professional life coaches—you'll see how personal and varied they can be.

- My Life Purpose is "to bring out the spirit in others," which also translates to "bringing out the passion or reigniting the passion in others." —*Merrily Sable*
- My life purpose is to be a mirror that reflects the brilliance and vibrancy of others back onto them, so that they can embrace their own purpose with the same sense of joy and reverie as I do mine. —*Kathleen O'Grady*

- My life purpose is to *feel great,* realizing confidently my unique and strong spirit, creating a comfortable place and a sense of family, giving intuitively to others. —*Kathleen Stanhope*
- My purpose in life is to inspire personal and spiritual growth, share my creative ideas, and connect meaningfully from the heart. —*Vicki Escude*
- My purpose is to live creatively and productively, without restrictions, while interacting with dynamic friends and colleagues, and consciously making decisions about my life choices. —*Gerri Vereen*
- My purpose is to passionately connect, excitedly perform, and creatively lead! —*Kathleen Mercker*
- My life purpose is to passionately seek, and enthusiastically share, secrets of creative collaboration. —*Jill Davis*
- I am most fulfilled when I am *fully present,* with my heart and my mind, *giving with purpose,* and *being valued,* to feel *connected, vibrant,* and at *peace.* — *Barb Patterson*

From a different view, our poet Shelby said, "As a retired teacher, I'm just now experiencing the joy of little granddaughters, discovering a gift for verse, adding new friends, and hoping to always listen to that inner voice 'people matter, not things.' "

You may not know exactly what these statements mean on a practical level, but each woman does. Create your own statement without worrying whether it's the correct format. If it feels right to you and will guide your decisions, live with it. It may serve you well for years, or, like me, you may change it unexpectedly in a moment of illumination.

Examples of manifesting your purpose

My coaching friend Merrily Sable wrote me, "Since I discovered my life purpose, I realize I have been manifesting it in various ways throughout my life through cheerleading, nursing, life coaching, mothering, etc. Your purpose does not change in life, but the manifestation of it shows up differently over time or with the seasons of your life."

That held true for Shelby, who shared a story about starting a ministry in her church. "I had never done anything like this. I started a ministry. Just myself. I got in front of the congregation and convinced them to help pick up this little boy and drive him to church. I said, 'This child loves coming here to church; he's learning about God. Do we really not want to pick him up on Sunday?' That poured out of me, just like the writing. It was a new experience. I'd never done anything like that before." Surprised though she was, Shelby's behavior was totally congruent with her values and her statement that "people matter, not things."

Kathleen gives expression to her purpose by writing books and articles, conducting seminars or giving speeches, and in her choice of volunteer activities. I teach traditional and online classes, coach individual clients, mentor young women, and serve as a role model to women of all ages. Our individual purposes combined to provide the guidelines for this book and are reflected clearly in the title *Second Blooming for Women: Growing a Life That Matters after Fifty.*

In what ways do you already manifest your life purpose? Are there other avenues for you to do so?

You have reached the final stage of this process and are now ready to craft an action plan for your *Second Blooming.*

Your action plan

Are you feeling a little overwhelmed thinking about an action plan for the rest of your life? Don't worry. It will develop step-by-step and will serve as your trusted guide through the coming years. As a fortune cookie message said, "You don't have to be perfect to fulfill your dreams." How true. You don't have to be perfect; you only have to be passionate, focused, and conscientious. Just as it takes time for a garden to mature, so does it take time for your *Second Blooming* plan to develop and come to fruition.

Frustrated one day at how long it was taking to write this book, Kathleen remarked to Shelby, "I can't believe we've been working on this for three whole years!" Shelby wisely replied, "Those three years would have passed anyway, and now look what you'll have to show for them." And so it will be for you. Persist, and over time, your accomplishments will accumulate.

You have already taken the first step in creating your action plan by establishing your goals. Think about the following questions:
- What are the tasks or functions involved in meeting each of my goals?
- What action steps do I need to take to accomplish the tasks?
- What resources (physical and mental) will I require to meet my goals?

Be prepared

Marcia Wieder, author of *Making Your Dreams Come True,* lists friends, friends of friends, family, and organizations or businesses as a few of her resources.[2] Other resources can include books, workshops, book clubs, discussion groups, time, training, and hobbies. Which resources are available to you?

Also consider what obstacles (those pesky weeds) are in your way. Wieder identifies "limiting beliefs" as barriers to achieving your dream; they are those conscious or subconscious things that you believe about yourself that hinder your ability to succeed[3] (e.g., I'm too old. It'll take too long. My husband won't support me. I'm not strong enough.). Other hurdles might include unsupportive friends, budget constraints, location, etc. Barriers don't necessarily indicate that you cannot or will not succeed, but they are issues for you to overcome as you grow toward living a life that matters. Do you know your obstructions? (Chapter 5 may provide assistance in overcoming some of them.) Staying focused on your goal will help keep you out of the weeds, too.

What is your timeline? Set one that is realistic and yet compels you to make progress. As mentioned previously, a timeline is meant to guide you, not increase your stress level. It's a part of the accountability plan, and the great thing is that, since you set it, you can change it. What is a realistic length of time to meet each of your goals? Establish your long-term target and then set short-term intervals toward that date.

How will you evaluate your progress toward accomplishing your goals? In my coaching practice, I ask my clients to rate their current status or progress on a scale of one to ten, with ten being the highest, and to state what they want their status to be in six months. They stay accountable because we have weekly check-in calls and they report their progress. How will you hold yourself accountable? Will you evaluate your progress daily, weekly, or monthly? With whom? How?

Wieder coaches her clients to create their "Dream Team," a group of friends who will support them in their quest to achieving their dream.[4] You, too, can create your own team, a "garden club" of supportive people. Can you identify three friends who will consistently bolster you on this venture? Or would you prefer to have an accountability partner or a life coach?

Your answers to these questions form the basis for your action plan. As you worked through this book, you gleaned all the tools and information required for a dynamic action plan. You're ready.

Creating an action plan

Here's an example of how the initial steps of my own plan would look. You can also find a blank form on our Web site at www.secondbloomingforwomen.com.

Betsy's Action Plan

My life purpose is to teach people how to discover their strengths and help them reach their dreams.

One way I can manifest my life purpose is to guide older women in living full, productive lives.

My goal is to write a book for women over fifty that coaches them in growing a life that matters.

Action Steps	Resources	Obstacles	Timelines	Accountability
1. Review books like ours, assess the competition, and find our niche.	Bookstores, libraries, Internet	Time, other projects	Complete review in three months.	Meet with or phone Kathleen every Tuesday at 2:00 p.m.
2. Brainstorm topics that the book should cover.	Presentations we've given, articles we've written	Finding the presentations, too many issues to choose from.	Two hours with follow up if necessary	Schedule appointment and reserve a room.
3. Outline chapters.	Books about writing a book proposal	Several books to choose from Which is best?	Complete one outline every week.	Share progress with the writers' group.
4.				
5.				
6.				

Now it's your turn. Take one logical step at a time. You can revise it as necessary.

My Action Plan

My life purpose _____

_____

One way I can manifest my life purpose _____

_____

My goal _____

_____

Action Steps	Resources	Obstacles	Timelines	Accountability

Techniques to ensure success

1. Visualization. Simply stated, visualization is *seeing* your success in your mind's eye. Competitive athletes, among others, use visualization. Have you noticed Olympic gymnasts as they wait for their turn to compete? As they pace the outer area of the venue, they go over their routine in their mind again and again. You can see their body making subtle moves that are, in actuality, their competitive routine. Golfers take their practice swings, visualizing the flight and the landing of the ball. Tennis players walk around practicing their serve as they wait for their match. Visualization is a powerful tool to use in accomplishing dreams. If you can see it, you can do it.

One of coach Dona's high school golf students reported that on the sixteenth hole in a tournament, she had her best score ever. If she had continued to play consistently through holes seventeen and eighteen, she would have had the best score of her life. However, she played the last two holes poorly, which kept her score average. Dona instructed the girl to do the following visualization in her next competition: "Write down your perfect score and draw a circle around it. Be certain that the circle is closed. The picture is clear, the score cannot escape, nor can anything get into the circle to affect it. Your subconscious can only see the perfect score." This was a powerful visualization. The girl complied— and won.

Find a quiet, comfortable, familiar place to practice your visualizations. It might be your favorite chair or your favorite spot at the park or beach. Give your full attention to your visualization and it will assist you in moving forward purposefully.

2. Law of Attraction. The Law of Attraction takes affirmations to the next level by asserting that people's thoughts (both conscious and unconscious) prescribe the reality of their lives, whether they're aware of it or not. Essentially, if you really want something and truly believe it's possible, you'll get it. Lynn Grabhorn's book, *Excuse Me, Your Life is Waiting,* presents her premise that everything in this world is made of energy— people, rocks, tables, and even blades of grass.[5] Physicists agree that energy and matter are the same; therefore, everything vibrates. Grabhorn credits feelings for the magnetic vibration from humans. According to her, when we are filled with joy, our emotions send out high frequency vibrations. When we are experiencing fear or worry, our vibrations are low frequencies. You are like a magnet attracting different kinds of people and experiences, like bees are attracted to nectar. What are you attracting? Are you vibrating at a high or low frequency?

3. Affirmations. Affirmations, too, play a vital role in achieving your dreams. An affirmation is a scripted, positive thought that you integrate into your life; it becomes a part of your thought process by being absorbed into your sub-conscious. Affirmations are positive, stated in the present tense, and repeated several times a day. Here are some sample affirmations for *Second Blooming* women:
- *I love and appreciate myself as I am.*
- *My life is blossoming bountifully.*
- *All things are working for good in my life.*
- *I am healthy and strong.*
- *My life's garden is beautiful.*
- *I am completely capable of reaching my goals.*

Choose an affirmation, or write one of your own, and read it aloud five times. Then copy it on ten pieces of paper, placing them where you will see them many times a day—on the refrigerator door or the mirror in the bathroom, in the book you're currently reading, on the dash of your car, on the treadmill, etc. Be certain to have your affirmation at your bedside so that you can repeat it five times every morning when you first awake, and every night before you drift off to sleep. Continue this process for thirty-two days and you will see significant progress toward your dreams.

The promise of your life purpose

Now that you know your life purpose and have a plan to activate it, you will begin to notice opportunities for the future that you couldn't see before. Your ability to say yes to projects that you are passionate about and no to others will be greatly enhanced. Confidence and courage will emanate from you. Difficult decisions will become effortless. You are now ready for the rest of your life. Your garden is in full bloom, and it's time to celebrate.

ADDITIONAL RESOURCES

The Path: Creating Your Mission Statement for Work and for Life by Laurie Beth Jones.

Excuse Me, Your Life Is Waiting by Lynn Grabhorn.

Plumeria

The plumeria is native to Mexico, Central America, and Venezuela. It has spread to all tropical areas of the world, especially Hawaii, where it grows so abundantly that many people think it's indigenous there. The plumeria tree produces flowers ranging from yellow to pink, which are most fragrant at night to lure sphinx moths to pollinate them. Visitors to Hawaii are often met with a quintessential greeting of aloha, a plumeria lei, containing dozens of fresh flowers strung together and hung around one's neck. In the book *A Varanda do Frangipani (Under the Frangipani)* by Mozambican author Mia Couto, the shedding of the tree's flowers serves to mark the passage of time.

— *Wikipedia*

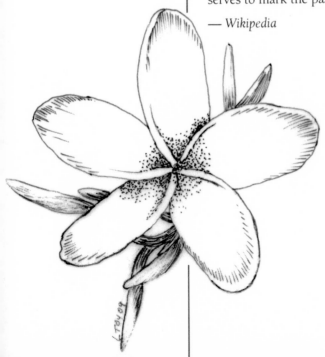

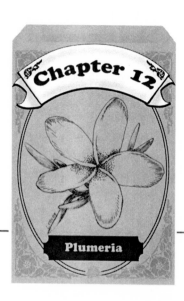

Chapter 12

Plumeria

Bloom!
Live a Life
That Matters

by Kathleen

*"To love what you do and feel that it matters—how could anything
be more fun?" ~ Katharine Graham*

You are uniquely beautiful, blooming brightly in the garden of life that
you have so thoughtfully envisioned and planted. Given all that you have
accomplished, you can consider yourself a master gardener.

Fate has given you this gift of bonus years. Honor, appreciate, and use
it by living from your heart and spirit. Always remember: whatever age
you are, it is the right age to start doing what you were called to do—your
purpose.

Expect the unexpected

After fifty, we seek meaning, authentic happiness, and a connection
to our common humanity. Just because living on purpose is the worthy
thing to do, though, doesn't mean it will always be easy. In any garden,
weeds constantly pop up and must be pulled, so be prepared.

One big challenge is living in a busy world with people expecting
you to be instantly accessible, whether by phone or e-mail, text message,
tweeting, or other means, and they often have urgent requests of you. But

are those requests important? Keep asking that critical question: *Is this important?* Multiple distractions can be increasingly hard to ignore as they tug on you, pulling you away from what's meaningful. Create some calm. Trust yourself. Center yourself. Be deliberate about how you live. What you do should bring you energy, joy, satisfaction, and a sense of value.

Every year, surprises sprout in your garden from seeds that have drifted in with the wind or been dropped by birds or squirrels, gracing you with their unexpected beauty. Likewise, you now have a purpose and an action plan, but seeds of possibility will inevitably interject themselves into your life, so always leave space for them to take root if they appeal to you.

Strive to live in all three realms that Seligman identified—pleasant, good, and meaningful—deploying your talents and signature strengths for the meaningful life. Aim for balance in these realms by making decisions and commitments consciously and thoughtfully.

Becoming role models

We talked early in the book about our society being a culture that values youth and evanescent beauty over experience, wisdom, and the lasting impact of valuable contributions. America, frankly, has a phobia about aging, but collectively we can change that shallow mind-set. The world's needs are too great and our individual gifts are too important to be devalued or dismissed. Young women will grow older, too, if they're lucky, and it's our job to be the role models for them that we did not have.

When the United States Navy commissions a new ship, it handpicks the crew, choosing the best people for each position because the precedents they set will establish the performance and reputation of the ship for decades. That first crew sets a standard of excellence which can help guarantee the future success of the ship and crew.

We are that inaugural crew for the *Second Blooming* stage of life, serving as role models for generations of women who will follow us. Younger women want to see a future worth anticipating, so they need us to inspire and motivate them, to be their leaders and guides, to set the bar high for a meaningful existence. By example, we can show them what authentic happiness is and how to grow a life that matters.

Women's stories

Since you heard from several women throughout this book, we thought you might be interested in knowing where they are in their *Second Blooming:*

Deb, fifty-two, estimates she has about five more years to work before she'll likely be required to retire. Although she doesn't have children of her own, she's very involved with her nephew. She especially liked the Growing Zones Chart, saying, "It rings true. I'm mostly in Zone 2, working towards Zone 3. That next phase is absolutely an exciting time. It offers freedom from work, especially the responsibilities of being boss. I anticipate fewer obligations and exploring the whole world on my own time frame, not while working ten-hour days. I want to uncover that passionate part, whatever it is." She's been married for twenty years.

Beth, fifty-seven, is a retired registered nurse. She says, "My *Second Blooming* started a couple years before I turned fifty. I stopped working when we moved here because of my husband's health. Now, ten years later, I have roots, where before, we were constantly traveling. What makes me happy? Writing, serving others, painting, feeling grounded." Beth volunteers with an adult literacy program, both as a tutor and a contributing writer to their newsletter. As opposed to two decades ago, "I'm free from responsibilities. I feel confident. My husband is surviving, and my heart is filled with gratitude." She and her husband have been married twenty-six years.

Maripaul, fifty-nine, was widowed when her son was one. Eventually she married the widowed father of one of her third-grade students. She volunteers at a museum where she started by composing handwritten notes to hundreds of contributors to whom thanks were overdue. Maripaul says, "The volunteering that works for me now allows me to learn and grow and stretch myself, and get back as well as give. It's not just giving of myself, but feeling good about myself and what I'm accomplishing." Her advice to others? "Find a niche where you're happy and they need you." She and her husband have been married for eighteen years.

Mary, sixty-one, feels at a standstill since her mother came to live with her. Although a full *Second Blooming* isn't possible right now, she continues her process of self-discovery through reading, teaching Sunday school classes, and taking the assessments identified in this book. Of her situation, she says, "I know I'm doing the right thing at the right time for the right reasons," and is content to wait her turn. After being divorced for several years, Mary and her second husband were introduced to each other by their daughters and have been married seventeen years. As you can imagine, the former teacher cherishes being a grandmother.

Shirley, sixty-three, says the biggest plus of this age is, "I have freedom now—physical, mental, and emotional. Because of the ages of my four children, I was a mother of kids for a long time. Now I'm able to do and discover things about myself that I didn't have time for when I was younger. I don't have so many obligations to fit into my day. Also, there's a deeper relationship with my friends. It's important to have a group to get some strength from." She reads all kinds of books and enjoys going to the movies—whenever she wants. She's been married for forty-three years and would love to become a grandmother.

Mamie, sixty-three, works full time at a university in the English Department where she instituted a "grammar hotline" for both students and the community. She's one of the few people we know for whom career, talents, passion, and purpose are perfectly matched. "I look forward to working on my next project," she says, "whatever it is. I will not go gently." Mamie finds, "Being old isn't bad, just an inconvenience. I keep working because it keeps me connected to the girl in me who still likes that career." She's single.

Shelby, sixty-nine, seemed to burst into bloom in the short time we've known her. She can put more meaning into fewer words than anyone we know, as you've seen in the poems she wrote for us. She's venturing out with her writing, submitting a piece to *AARP*, and entering a poetry contest. "I relish what I'm learning about myself," she said. "I'm still getting surprises and new insights about myself, some painful, but I'm still growing. New opportunities come to me out of the blue. Like this book. It's been a nice journey to go along with you." Shelby and her husband have been married forty-seven years, and are enjoying their two grandchildren.

Anne, eighty-five, continues to paint in an upstairs studio at home, generously donating her skills when a project touches her heart. Her son-in-law helps sell her work through a gallery in Ohio, and belonging to a local co-op art gallery "motivates me to do more." Trips to Europe combine her faith, love of churches, and talent in beautiful watercolors of cathedrals. "While painting, I can lose myself. It's the only thing I do that can make me forget to eat." For Anne, "The reward is here on earth in the way you live and relate to people." She and her husband celebrated sixty-two years of marriage.

Reflection

You've come a long way since beginning this book, living purposefully and passionately, with values, vision, goals, and activities aligned to the best of your ability. You have cultivated your *Second Blooming* by using your talents, strengths, and skills for a purposeful life. Now it's time for reflection. Contemplate the following topics, preferably in your journal so you can refer back to your thoughts later. You can print the questions at www.secondbloomingforwomen.com.

• What have you accomplished since starting *Second Blooming*? What progress have you made toward your vision?

• In your opinion, what roles do passion, dreams, and purpose play in the lives of women over fifty?

• What were some of your feelings along the way (e.g., fear, surprise, excitement, intimidation, relief, joy)?

• Did you hit any roadblocks? What were they and how did you get past them?

• Which people were helpful; what did they do? Who was not helpful and in what way?

• What important lessons did you learn about yourself or life in general?

• Has your self-image changed since starting the book? If so, how?

• In what ways, large and small, does your life matter? What are you doing that's making a positive difference?

Celebrate! And keep blooming, wherever you plant yourself.

A smile radiates
As I view this garden
As I view my life
Always changing
Ah, sweet fragrance
We are both beautiful
Regardless of the passing seasons.
~ Shelby Miller

ACTIVITY

Please share your Second Blooming experiences or stories with us and other women at www.secondbloomingforwomen.com.

ABOUT THE AUTHORS

Kathleen Vestal Logan, M.S., M.A.

In a seemingly peripatetic life, Kathleen Logan has been an elementary school teacher, naval officer, writer and speaker on navy deployments and family life, counselor, college instructor, and coordinator of a hospital-based employee assistance program. Currently, she does private consulting. She has conducted hundreds of lively seminars for businesses, civic organizations, and nonprofit groups on building personal skills and enhancing relationships. She inspires and empowers people to trust themselves while developing a vision for their future. Married to a career naval officer, Kathleen and their son moved frequently and experienced long separations. With each new duty station or deployment, she had to reach deep inside herself to find personal resources to help her not just adapt, but thrive, in changing circumstances.

Kathleen has had articles published in the U.S. Naval Institute magazine, *Proceedings*, and *Toastmaster Magazine*. She has a bachelor's degree in education, a master's degree in management, and a master's degree in marriage and family therapy.

E. L. (Betsy) Smith, Ph.D.

Betsy's two top strengths are strategic (innovative, original, and resourceful) and maximizer (has a keen ability to help people embrace and savor their success). A proud Texas Aggie, Betsy is a certified professional life coach. Her highly developed sense of humor combined with her boundless energy and her zest for life create her coaching style—fast-paced, bold, purposeful with great results, and, of course, fun!

Betsy has a bachelor's degree in psychology and social work, a master's degree in adult education, and a Ph.D. in higher education administration. She was recognized as one of the thirty distinguished graduates from the College of Education at Texas A&M University. Her long and extraordinary career at a large community college in Pensacola, Florida, involved coaching female students, faculty, and staff to greater self-confidence and success. She has had articles published in both magazines and academic journals, and is a well-known speaker and seminar leader.

Kathleen and Betsy co-authored articles on "Second Blooming for Women" published in *On the Coast Magazine* and *Coming of Age: Lifestyle Magazine for Seniors*. The latter article was awarded bronze in the 2009 National Mature Media Awards competition. They are both enjoying their own *Second Blooming*.

ACKNOWLEDGMENTS

We are grateful to our many friends and colleagues who contributed to *Second Blooming.*

Thank you to our writers' group, Write On! Pensacola, which has been with us from the inception of this project. Their encouragement and input kept us enthused and focused. We deeply appreciate the countless hours that Mary Blanchard, Barbara McCarren, and Mary Beth Sloan spent reviewing the chapters, and are thankful for their insight and invaluable feedback.

Jeff Nall, editor of Council on Aging of West Florida's *Coming of Age* magazine, published our article "Second Blooming for Women" in 2008. He continues to share his knowledge of marketing and publicity with us.

Special thanks to Lyda Toy for her original and exquisite flower sketches introducing each chapter. Derek Ferebee provided the stunning flower photography for the cover as well as technical assistance in transmitting Lyda's sketches and his photos to our publisher. We also appreciate Rob Engel, Kris Thoma, and Jackie Scrimpshire who shared their computer expertise when we were stumped.

Karyn Engle, our virtual assistant, receives recognition for assembling separate computer files into one file, "The Book," when our efforts to do so scrambled the formatting of everything. Kathy Lee Coker, thank you for the early grammatical editing.

We were elated the day publisher Nancy Cleary said, "I love, love, love your proposal," and took us on as clients. She has been a wonderful cheerleader and a source of essential information ever since. The clever "seed packet" book cover was her design.

Extra thanks go to our beloved husbands, C. Flack Logan and Jack Parkin, for their patience, confidence, and essential support during this longer-than-expected venture.

And how do we possibly express our profound gratitude to the women of the book—Deb, Beth, Maripaul, Mary, Shirley, Mamie, Shelby, and Anne—who were so generous with both their time and spirit? Their thoughtfulness and soul-searching honesty enriched everything we wrote, helping all of us to understand ourselves, our challenges, and our opportunities in a deeper, more meaningful way.

Finally, thank you to the countless, wonderful women who believed in what we were writing and kept us motivated by asking, "How's the book coming?" May we all thrive and live lives that matter in our *Second Blooming*.

ENDNOTES

Epigraph: Agatha Christie, *An Autobiography* (New York: Dodd, Mead & Company, 1977), 507.

Introduction
1. Gail Sheehy, *New Passages: Mapping Your Life across Time* (New York: Random House, 1995), 16.
2. Sue Shellenbarger, *The Breaking Point: How Female Midlife Crisis Is Transforming Today's Woman* (New York: Henry Holt, 2004), 66.
3. Suzanne Braun Levine, *Inventing the Rest of Our Lives: Women in Second Adulthood* (New York: Penguin Group Plume Press, 2006), 5.
4. Sara Davidson, *Leap! What Will We Do with the Rest of Our Lives?* (New York: Random House, 2007), 9.

Chapter 1: History Sows the Seeds for Women's Second Blooming
Quote: Gail Sheehy, *New Passages: Mapping Your Life across Time* (New York: Random House, 1995), 4.
1. "The History of Women's Suffrage," http://www.history.com/minisite.do?content_type=Minisite_Generic&content_type_id=93 (accessed January 26, 2009).
2. E. Susan Barber, "One Hundred Years toward Suffrage: An Overview," *National American Woman Suffrage Association Collection Home Page,* http://memory.loc.gov/ammem/naw/nawstime.html (accessed January 26, 2009).
3. Barber, "One Hundred Years toward Suffrage: An Overview."
4. History.com, "The History of Women's Suffrage."
5. History.com, "The History of Women's Suffrage."
6. Barber, "One Hundred Years toward Suffrage: An Overview."
7. Barber, "One Hundred Years toward Suffrage: An Overview."
8. "The Birth Control Pill Celebrates Forty Years of Fame," May 8, 2000, http://www.riskworld.com/PressRel/2000/00q2/PR00a129.htm (accessed January 22, 2009).
9. Sandy Cohen, "Birth control pills helped empower women, changed the world," *Copley News Service,* July 17, 2005, http://www.religiousconsultation.org/ News_Tracker/birth_control_pills_helped_empower_ (accessed 22 January 2009).
10. "Timeline: The Pill," *American Experience,* http://www.pbs.org/wgbh/amex/pill/timeline/timeline2.html (accessed January 30, 2007).
11. "Timeline: The Pill."
12. "Timeline: The Pill."
13. "Timeline: The Pill."
14. "Timeline: The Pill."
15. Cohen, "Birth control pills helped empower women, changed the world."

16. Mark Coultan, "Feminist icon Betty Friedan dies on her birthday," February 6, 2006, *The Age Company Ltd.*, http://www.theage.com.au/news/world/feminist-icon-betty-friedan-dies-on-her-birthday/20 (accessed January 22, 2009).

17. Betty Friedan, *The Feminine Mystique* (New York: W. W. Norton & Company, Inc., 1997), 525. The book was originally published in 1963.

18. Margalit Fox, "Betty Friedan, Who Ignited Cause in 'Feminine Mystique,' Dies at 85," *New York Times*, February 4, 2006, http://www.nytimes.com/2006/02/04/national/05cnd-friedan.html?r=1 (accessed January 22, 2009).

19. "Civil Rights Act of 1964–New World Encyclopedia," *Info:Main Page–New World Encyclopedia,* http://www.newworldencyclopedia.org/entry/Civil_Rights_Act_of_1964 (accessed January 27, 2009).

20. "Civil Rights Act United States 1964–Britannica Online Encyclopedia," *Encyclopedia - Britannica Online Encyclopedia,* http://www.britannica.com/EBchecked/topic/ 119351/Civil-Rights-Act?view=print (accessed January 27, 2009).

21. "Civil Rights Act of 1964–New World Encyclopedia."

22. "The Civil Rights Act of 1964." *AFRICANAMERICANS.com.* http://www.africanamericans.com/CivilRightsActof1964.htm (accessed January 27, 2009).

23. Jill Lieber Steeg, "Lawsuits, disputes reflect continuing tension over Title IX," *USA Today,* May 13, 2008, Sec. A: 1.

24. Steeg, "Lawsuits, disputes reflect continuing tension over Title IX."

25. "What Is Title IX?" *Welcome to American University, Washington, DC USA,* http://www.american.edu/sadker/titleix.htm (accessed January 30, 2007).

26. Kathy Gill, "Issue Summary: Abortion," *About.com US Politics,* http://uspolitics.about.com/od/electionissues/i/abortion.htm (accessed January 27, 2009).

27. Gill, "Issue Summary: Abortion."

28. Gill, "Issue Summary: Abortion."

Chapter 2: Climate Map: Thrive in Your Natural Growing Zone

Quote: Adrienne Rich, *Of Woman Born: Motherhood As Experience and Institution* (New York: Bantam Books, 1997), 150.

1. Chris Crowley and Henry S. Lodge, M.D., *Younger Next Year* (New York: Workman Publishing Company, Inc., 2004), xxxii.

2. Crowley and Lodge, *Younger Next Year,* 6.

Chapter 3: Aeration: Loosen the Soil of Your Attitude

Quote: Martha Washington, *The Critic* (New York: The Critic Company, January-June 1897, vol. xxvii), 87.

1. Martin E. P. Seligman, Ph.D., *Authentic Happiness* (New York: Free Press, 2002), 15.

2. Marilyn Elias, "Psychologists Now Know What Makes People Happy," *USA Today*, December 10, 2002, http://www.usatoday.com/news/health/2002-12-08-happy-main_x.html (accessed February 8, 2009).
3. Becca R. Levy and others, "Longevity Increased by Positive Self-Perceptions of Aging," *Journal of Personality and Social Psychology*, vol. 83, no. 2 (2002): 265.
4. James D'Angelo, "The Healing Power of the Human Voice," *Pensacola News Journal*, August 28, 2007, Sec. B: 1.
5. Dr. Lee Burk and Dr. Stanley Tan, "Therapeutic Benefits of Laughter," http://www.holistic-online.com/humor_therapy/humor_therapy_benefits.html (accessed March 2, 2009).
6. Burk and Tan, "Therapeutic Benefits of Laughter."
7. American Music Therapist Association, "Frequently Asked Questions," http://www.musictherapy.org/faqs.html (accessed March 4, 2009).
8. Robert A. Emmons and Michael E. McCullough, "Highlights from the Research Project on Gratitude and Thankfulness, Dimensions and Perspectives of Gratitude," http://www.psychology.ucdavis.edu/labs/emmons (accessed March 4, 2009).

Chapter 4: Are You Root Bound? Embrace Change

Quote: Gail Sheehy, *New Passages: Mapping Your Life across Time* (New York: Random House, 1995), 148.
1. Gregory Mitchell, "Carl Jung and Jungian Analytical Psychology," http://www.trans4mind.com/mind-development/jung.html (accessed August 28, 2009).
2. Mitchell, "Carl Jung and Jungian Analytical Psychology."
3. Erik Erikson, *Childhood and Society* (New York: W. W. Norton & Company, 1950), 231.
4. Erikson, *Childhood and Society,* 231-233.
5. Stephen R. Covey, *The 7 Habits of Highly Effective People* (New York: Fireside, 1989), 81-85.

Chapter 5: Weeds: Pull Them to Improve Your Life's Yield

Quote: William Shakespeare, *Macbeth,* Act 5, Scene 1.
1. Gabrielle deGroot Redford, "Get off the couch! Surefire tips for sticking to your resolution to get more exercise," *AARP The Magazine* (January & February 2008), 27.
2. Redford, "Get off the couch!" 27.
3. Candis Reade, "Statistics on Spousal Abuse," http://ezinearticles.com/?statistics-on-spousal-abuse&id=1578447 (accessed May 1, 2009).
4. Christianne Northrup, *Women's Bodies, Women's Wisdom* (New York: Bantam Books, 1998), 8.
5. Sandra Block, Your Money, "Husbands should consider delaying Social Security benefits," *USA Today,* January 15, 2008, Sec. B.

6. F. John Reh, "Pareto's Principle—The 80–20 Rule," *About.com Management*, http://management.about.com/cs/generalmanagement/a/Pareto081202.htm?p=1 (accessed March 16, 2009).

7. *Random House Webster's College Dictionary*, "worry," 1094.

Chapter 6: Organics: Trust Your Authentic Self

Quote: Sue Patton Thoele, *Growing Hope: Seeds of Positive Change in Your Life and in the World* (York Beach, Maine: Conari Press, 2004), 190.

1. Wayne Dyer, Ph. D., *There's a Spiritual Solution to Every Problem* (New York: HarperCollins Publishers, 2001), 2.

2. Dyer, *There's a Spiritual Solution to Every Problem*, 9.

3. Dyer, *There's a Spiritual Solution to Every Problem*, 14.

4. Arlene F. Harder, "Erik Erikson's Stages of Psychosocial Development," http://www.support4change.com/stages/cycles/Erikson.html (accessed March 3, 2009).

5. Robert Needleman, "Birth Order: The Basics," http://www.drspock.com/article/0,1510,5550,00.html (accessed October 12, 2008).

6. Needleman, "Birth Order: The Basics."

Chapter 7: Perennials: Appreciate Who You Are

Quote: Marilyn Zelinsky, *The Inspired Workspace: Designs for Creativity and Productivity* (Gloucester, Massachusetts: Rockport Publishers, 2002), 141.

1. David Keirsey, Ph.D., *Please Understand Me II* (Del Mar, California: Prometheus Nemesis Book Company, 1998), 20-26.

2. Marcus Buckingham and Donald O. Clifton, Ph.D., *Now, Discover Your Strengths* (New York: Free Press, 2001), 29.

3. Martin E. P. Seligman, Ph.D., *Authentic Happiness* (New York: Free Press, 2002), 134-137.

4. Seligman, *Authentic Happiness*, 47.

5. Marcus Buckingham, *Go Put Your Strengths to Work* (New York: Free Press, 2007), 43.

6. Buckingham, *Go Put Your Strengths to Work*, 49.

7. "KTS-The Keirsey Temperament Sorter (KTS-II)," *Keirsey.com*, http://www.keirsey.com/aboutkts2.aspx (accessed August 4, 2008).

8. "About 4 Temperaments: The Guardians," *Keirsey.com*, http://www.keirsey.com/handler.aspx?s=keirsey&f=fourtemps&tab=4&c=overview (accessed August 4, 2008).

9. "KTS-II CLASSIC Temperament Report," 2, *Keirsey.com*, Advisorteam, a division of Keirsey.com, http://www.keirsey.com/sorter/user.aspx (accessed August 4, 2008). This report is only available when character subtype is purchased.

10. "About 4 Temperaments - The Idealists." *Keirsey.com*, http://www.keirsey.com/handler.aspx?s=keirsey&f=fourtemps&tab=4&c=overview (accessed August 4, 2008).

11. "About 4 Temperaments - The Rationals," *Keirsey.com*, http://www.keirsey.com/handler.aspx?s=keirsey&f=fourtemps&tab=4&c=overview (accessed August 4, 2008).
12. "KTS-II CLASSIC Temperament Report," 10.
13. "KTS-II CLASSIC Temperament Report," 19.
14. Seligman, *Authentic Happiness*, 134.
15. Buckingham and Clifton, *Now, Discover Your Strengths*, 29.
16. Buckingham and Clifton, *Now, Discover Your Strengths*, 11-13.
17. Buckingham and Clifton, *Now, Discover Your Strengths*, 111.
18. Buckingham and Clifton, *Now, Discover Your Strengths*, 106.
19. Buckingham and Clifton, *Now, Discover Your Strengths*, 108.
20. Buckingham and Clifton, *Now, Discover Your Strengths*, 245.
21. Buckingham and Clifton, *Now, Discover Your Strengths*, 78-79.
22. Claudia Wallis, "The New Science of Happiness," *Time Magazine*, January 17, 2005, http://www.authentichappiness.sas.upenn.edu/images/TimeMagazine/Time-Happiness.pdf (accessed March 30, 2009).
23. Seligman, *Authentic Happiness*, 260-263.
24. Buckingham, *Go Put Your Strengths to Work*, 53.
25. Buckingham, *Go Put Your Strengths to Work*, 69.
26. Seligman, *Authentic Happiness*, 13.

Chapter 8: Annuals: Inventory Your Skills

Quote: Anne Wilson Schaef, *Meditations for People Who (may) Worry Too Much* (New York: Random House, 1996), 14.
1. Marcus Buckingham, *Go Put Your Strengths to Work* (New York: Free Press, 2007), 75.
2. "Skills Identification—Skills," 1, Minnesota Department of Employment and Economic Development, http://www.deed.state.mn.us/cjs/cjsbook/skills1.htm (accessed April 14, 2009).
3. "Finding a Job with Skills You Already Have," 2, Connecticut Department of Labor. http://www.ctdol.state.ct.us/progsupt/jobsrvce/skills.htm (accessed April 14, 2009).
4. "Finding a Job with Skills You Already Have," 3.
5. Marcus Buckingham and Donald O. Clifton, Ph.D., *Now, Discover Your Strengths* (New York: Free Press, 2001), 46.

Chapter 9: Decide What to Plant: Clarify Your Passions and Dreams

Quote: James Miller, *Visions from Earth* (Victoria, B.C., Canada: Trafford Publishing, 2004), 132.
1. Jane Hess Collins, "Transformative Travel: Volunteering changed her world," *USA Today*, January 2, 2009, Sec. D: 1.
2. Barbara Sher, *It's Only Too Late If You Don't Start Now* (New York: Dell Publishing, 1998), 319.
3. Shannon Lord, "Make-A-Wish Foundation." *Pensacola Today* (February & March 2004), 50.

4. Rev. Nan Adams, "The Myth of Scarcity."

5. *Random House Webster's College Dictionary,* "passion," 968.

6. Sheri McConnell, *The Woman's Book of Powerful Quotations* (Kearney, Nebraska: Morris Publishing, 2006), 177.

7. *Random House Webster's College Dictionary,* "dream," 401.

8. Donna Freckmann, "Hooked on a feeling," *Pensacola News Journal*, April 10, 2008, Sec. B: 1.

Chapter 10: Pinch and Prune: Ascertain Your Values and Vision

Quote: Karen Casey, *Every Day a New Beginning: A Meditation Book and Journal for Daily Reflections* (Center City, Minnesota: Hazelden Publishing, 2001), 16.

1. S. H. Schwartz, "Universals in the Context and Structure of Values: Theoretical Advances and Empirical Test in 20 Countries," *Advances in Experimental Social Psychology*, M. Zanna, ed., (San Diego: Academic Press, 1992), 1002.

2. Harriett Braiker, *The Disease to Please: Curing the People-Pleasing Syndrome* (New York: McGraw Hill, 2001), xi.

3. Judith Tingley, "No, No and No Again," *Toastmaster Magazine*, vol. 70, No. 9 (September 2004), 24.

4. Rosabeth Moss Kanter, *Evolve: Succeeding in the Digital Culture of Tomorrow* (Watertown, Massachusetts: Harvard Business Press, 2001), 264.

5. Laurie Beth Jones, *The Path: Creating Your Mission Statement for Work and for Life* (New York: Hyperion, 1996), 73-75.

6. Jones, *The Path*, 73.

7. Jones, *The Path*, 79.

8. Jim Collins, *Good to Great* (New York: Harper Collins Publishers, 2001), 197.

9. Dena Harris, "Set SMART Goals for Speaking Progress," *Toastmaster Magazine* vol. 74, No. 9 (September 2008), 24.

10. Sara Reistad-Long, "If You Need A Push…," *O The Oprah Magazine,* vol. 9, Issue 9 (September 2008), 208.

11. Harris, "Set SMART Goals for Speaking Progress," 24.

12. Jennifer Sturz Ratna, "Life Coaching," www.coaching-essence.com/about-coaching (accessed March 8, 2009).

Chapter 11: Add Water, Fertilizer, and Sunshine: Bring Your Purpose to Life with a Plan

Quote: John Cook, Steve Deger, and Leslie Ann Gibson, *The Book of Positive Quotations,* 2nd ed., (Minneapolis, Minnesota: Fairview Press, 2007), 556.

1. Laurie Beth Jones, *The Path: Creating Your Mission Statement for Work and for Life* (New York: Hyperion, 1996), 63.

2. Marcia Wieder, *Making Your Dreams Come True* (New York: Harmony Books, 1993), 148.

3. Wieder, *Making Your Dreams Come True*, 94.

4. Wieder, *Making Your Dreams Come True*, 220.

Chapter 12: Bloom! Live a Life that Matters
Quote: Genevieve Brown and Beverly J. Irby, *Women and Leadership: Creating Balance in Life* (Hauppauge, New York: Nova Publishers, 2001), 43.

BIBLIOGRAPHY

Adams, John D., and Sabina A. Spencer. *Life Changes: Growing through Personal Transitions.* San Luis Obispo, California: Impact Publishers, 1990.

Adams, Rev. Nan M. "The Myth of Scarcity: God's Utterly Reliable Abundance." Sermon delivered at Trinity Presbyterian Church, Pensacola, Florida, July 29, 2007.

Alspaugh, Nancy, and Marilyn Kentz. *Not Your Mother's Mid-Life: A Ten-Step Guide to Fearless Aging.* Kansas City, Missouri: Andrews McMeel Publishing, 2003.

Anderson, Joan. *The Second Journey: The Road Back to Yourself.* New York: Hyperion, 2008.

Baar, Karen. *For My Next Act: Women Scripting Life after 50.* New York: St. Martin's Press, 2004.

Barletta, Marti. *Primetime for Women: How to Win the Hearts, Minds, and Business of Boomer Big Spenders.* Chicago, Illinois: Kaplan Publishing, 2007.

Belf, Teri-E. *Coaching with Spirit: Allowing Success to Emerge.* San Francisco, California: Jossey-Bass/Pfeiffer, 2002.

Beaman, Rhonda, Ed.D. *You're Only Young Twice: 10 Do-Overs to Reawaken Your Spirit.* Acton, Massachusetts: Vanderwyk & Burnham, 2006.

Bender, Steve, ed. *The Southern Living Garden Book.* Birmingham, Alabama: Oxmoor House, Inc., 1998.

Blair, Pamela D., Ph.D. *The Next Fifty Years: A Guide for Women at Midlife and Beyond.* Charlottesville, Virginia: Hampton Roads Publishing Company, 2005.

Braiker, Harriett. *The Disease to Please: Curing the People-Pleasing Syndrome.* New York: McGraw Hill, 2001.

Breathnach, Sarah Ban. *Simple Abundance: A Day Book of Comfort and Care.* New York: Warner Books, 1995.

Brown, Genevieve and Beverly J. Irby. *Women and Leadership: Creating Balance in Life.* Hauppauge, New York: Nova Publishers, 2001.

Buckingham, Marcus, and Donald O. Clifton, Ph.D. *Now, Discover Your Strengths.* New York: Free Press, 2001.

Buckingham, Marcus. *Go Put Your Strengths to Work: 6 Powerful Steps to Achieve Outstanding Performance.* New York: Free Press, 2007.

Casey, Karen. *Each Day a New Beginning: A Meditation Book and Journal for Daily Reflection.* Center City, Minnesota: Hazelden Publishing, 2001.

Christie, Agatha. *An Autobiography.* New York: Dodd, Mead & Company, 1977.

Collins, Jim. *Good to Great: Why Some Companies Make the Leap…and Others Don't.* New York: HarperCollins, 2001.

Cook, John, Steve Deger, and Leslie Ann Gibson. *The Book of Positive Quotations*, 2nd ed. Minneapolis, Minnesota: Fairview Press, 2007.

Covey, Stephen R. *The 7 Habits of Highly Effective People: Powerful Lessons in Personal Change.* New York: Fireside, 1989.

Crowley, Chris, and Henry S. Lodge, M.D. *Younger Next Year for Women: Live Strong, Fit, and Sexy—Until You're 80 and Beyond.* New York: Workman Publishing Company, Inc., 2004.

Davidson, Sara. *LEAP! What Will We Do with the Rest of Our Lives?* New York: Random House, 2007.

De Angelis, Barbara, Ph.D. *Secrets about Life Every Woman Should Know: Ten Principles for Total Emotional and Spiritual Fulfillment.* New York: Hyperion, 1999.

Downing, Colette. *Red Hot Mamas: Coming Into Our Own at Fifty.* New York: Bantam Books, 1997.

Duerk, Judith. *Circle of Stones: Woman's Journey to Herself.* Philadelphia, Pennsylvania: Innisfree Press, Inc., 1989.

Dyer, Wayne, Ph.D. *There's a Spiritual Solution to Every Problem.* New York: HarperCollins, 2001.

Erikson, Erik H. *Childhood and Society.* New York: W. W. Norton & Company, 1950.

Escude, Vicki. *Create Your Day with Intention! The Thirty Day Power Coach.* Asheville, North Carolina: Six-S Press, 2005.

Fisher, Renee, Jean Peelen, and Joyce Kramer. *Invisible No More: The Secret Lives of Women Over 50.* New York: iUniverse, 2005.

Friedan, Betty. *The Feminine Mystique.* New York: W. W. Norton & Company, Inc., 1997.

_____. *The Fountain of Age.* New York: Simon & Schuster, 1993.

Golden, C. J. *Tao of the Defiant Woman: Five Brazen Ways to Accept What You Must and Rebel Against the Rest.* Naperville, Illinois: Sourcebooks, Inc., 2007.

Grabhorn, Lynn. *Excuse Me, Your Life Is Waiting: The Astonishing Power of Feelings.* Charlottesville, Virginia: Hampton Roads Publishing Company, Inc., 2000.

Hall, Calvin S., and Gardner Lindzey. *Theories of Personality,* 2nd ed. New York: John Wiley & Sons, Inc., 1970.

Harris, Dena. "Set SMART Goals for Speaking Progress." *Toastmaster Magazine* (September 2008): 24-26.

Harris, Thomas A., M.D. *I'm OK – You're OK.* New York: HarperCollins Publishers, Inc., 1967.

Jacobs, Ruth Harriet, Ph.D. *Be an Outrageous Older Woman.* New York: Harper Perennial, 1997.

Johnson, Richard P., Ph.D. *The New Retirement: Discovering Your Dream.* St. Louis, Missouri: World Press, 2001.

Johnson, Spencer, M.D. *Who Moved My Cheese? An A-Mazing Way to Deal with Change in Your Work and in Your Life.* New York: G. P. Putnam's Sons, 1998.

Jones, Laurie Beth. *The Path: Creating Your Mission Statement for Work and for Life.* New York: Hyperion, 1996.

Kanter, Elizabeth Moss. *Evolve: Succeeding in the Digital Culture of Tomorrow.* Watertown, Massachusetts: Harvard Business Press, 2001.

Keirsey, David, Ph.D. *Please Understand Me II: Temperament, Character, Intelligence.* Del Mar, California: Prometheus Nemesis Book Company, 1998.

Levine, Suzanne Braun. *Inventing the Rest of Our Lives: Women in Second Adulthood.* New York: Penguin Group Plume Press, 2006.

Levy, Becca R., Martin D. Slade, Stanislav V. Kasl, and Suzanne R. Kunkel. "Longevity Increased by Positive Self-Perceptions of Aging." *Journal of Personality and Social Psychology*, vol. 83, No. 2, (2002): 265.

Lord, Shannon. "Make-A-Wish Foundation." *Pensacola Today* (February & March 2004): 50.

Marston, Stephanie. *If Not Now, When? Reclaiming Ourselves at Midlife.* New York: Warner Books, 2002.

McConnell, Sheri. *The Woman's Book of Powerful Quotations.* Kearney, Nebraska: Morris Publishing, 2006.

Miller, James. *Visions from Earth.* Victoria, B.C., Canada: Trafford Publishing, 2006.

Northrup, Christiane. *Women's Bodies, Women's Wisdom: Creating Physical and Emotional Health and Healing.* New York: Bantam Books, 1998.

Orman, Suze. *The 9 Steps to Financial Freedom: Practical and Spiritual Steps So You Can Stop Worrying.* New York: Crown Publishers, 1997.

Random House Webster's College Dictionary. New York: Random House, 2001.

Rath, Tom. *Strengths Finder 2.0: A New and Upgraded Edition of the Online Test from Gallup's Now, Discover Your Strengths.* New York: Gallup Press, 2007.

Redford, Gabrielle deGroot. "Get Off the Couch! Surefire tips for sticking to your resolution to get more exercise." *AARP The Magazine* (January & February 2008): 26-27.

Reistad-Long, Sara. "If You Need a Push." *O The Oprah Magazine* (September 2008): 208.

Rich, Adrienne. *Of Woman Born: Motherhood As Experience and Institution.* New York:Bantam Books, 1997.

Richardson, Carol. *The Art of Extreme Self Care.* Carlsbad, California: Hay House Publishers, 2009.

Rountree, Cathleen. *On Women Turning 50: Celebrating Mid-Life Discoveries.* New York: HarperCollins, 1993.

Schwartz, S. H., "Universals in the Context and Structure of Values: Theoretical Advances and Empirical Tests in 20 Countries." *Advances in Experimental Social Psychology.* M. Zanna, ed. San Diego, California: Academic Press, 1992.

Seligman, Martin E. P., Ph.D. *Authentic Happiness: Using the New Positive Psychology to Realize Your Potential for Lasting Fulfillment.* New York: Free Press, 2002.

Schaef, Anne Wilson, Ph.D. *Meditations for People Who (may) Worry Too Much.* New York: Random House, 1996.

Sheehy, Gail. *New Passages: Mapping Your Life across Time.* New York: Random House, 1995.

Shellenbarger Sue. *The Breaking Point: How Female Midlife Crisis Is Transforming Today's Woman.* New York: Henry Holt, 2004.

Sher, Barbara. *It's Only Too Late if You Don't Start Now: How to Create Your Second Life at Any Age.* New York: Dell Publishing, 1998.

St. James, Elaine. *Living the Simple Life: A Guide to Scaling Down and Enjoying More.* New York: Hyperion, 1996.

Swartz, Susan. *The Juicy Tomatoes Guide to Ripe Living after 50.* Oakland, California: New Harbinger Publications, 2006.

Tenneson, Joyce. *Wise Women: A Celebration of Their Insights, Courage, and Beauty.* Boston: Bullfinch Press, 2002.

Thoele, Sue Patton. *Growing Hope: Sowing the Seeds of Positive Change in Your Life and the World.* York Beach, Maine: Conari Press, 2004.

Tingley, Judith. "No, No and No Again." *Toastmaster Magazine* (September 2004): 22-24.

Wallis, Claudia, et al. "The New Science of Happiness." *Time Magazine,* January 17, 2005: 2-9.

Weaver, Frances. *Girls with the Grandmother Faces: A Celebration of Life's Potential for Those over 55.* New York: Hyperion, 1996.

Weiner-Davis, Michele. *Change Your Life and Everyone in It: How To.* New York: Simon and Schuster, 1996.

Wieder, Marcia. *Making Your Dreams Come True: A Plan for Easily Discovering and Achieving the Life You Want.* New York: Harmony Books, 1993.

Marilyn Zelinsky. *The Inspired Workspace: Designs for Creativity and Productivity.* Gloucester, Massachusetts: Rockport Publishers, 2004.